AF166256

The Mindful Qualitative Researcher

To Vera Lou Petersen

May her shortened life remind us to never take a single breath for granted.

As a global academic publisher, Sage is driven by the belief that research and education are critical in shaping society. Our mission is building bridges to knowledge—supporting the development of ideas into scholarship that is certified, taught, and applied in the real world.

Sage's founder, Sara Miller McCune, transferred control of the company to an independent trust, which guarantees our independence indefinitely. This enables us to support an equitable academic future over the long term by building lasting relationships, championing diverse perspectives, and co-creating social and behavioral science resources that transform teaching and learning.

The Mindful Qualitative Researcher

Laura L. Lemon

University of Alabama, Tuscaloosa

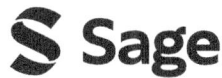

QUALITATIVE RESEARCH METHODS SERIES

Series Editor: David L. Morgan, Portland State University

The *Qualitative Research Methods Series* currently consists of 64 volumes that address essential aspects of using qualitative methods across social and behavioral sciences. These widely used books provide valuable resources for a broad range of scholars, researchers, teachers, students, and community-based researchers.

The series publishes volumes that:

- Address topics of current interest to the field of qualitative research.

- Provide practical guidance and assistance with collecting and analyzing qualitative data.

- Highlight essential issues in qualitative research, including strategies to address those issues.

- Add new voices to the field of qualitative research.

A key characteristic of the Qualitative Research Methods Series is an emphasis on both a *"why"* and a *"how-to"* perspective, so that readers will understand the purposes and motivations behind a method, as well as the practical and technical aspects of using that method. These relatively short and inexpensive books rely on a cross-disciplinary approach, and they typically include examples from practice; tables, boxes, and figures; discussion questions; application activities; and further reading sources.

New volumes in the Series include:

The Mindful Qualitative Researcher

Laura L. Lemon

Qualitative Research Writing: Credible and Trustworthy Writing from Beginning to End

Michelle Salmona, Dan Kaczynski, and Eli Lieber

Crafting Qualitative Research Questions

Elizabeth (Betsy) A. Baker

Narrative as Topic and Method in Social Research

Donileen R. Loseke

Introduction to Cognitive Ethnography and Systematic Field Work

G. Mark Schoepfle

Photovoice for Social Justice: Visual Representation in Action

Jean M. Breny and Shannon L. McMorrow

For information on how to submit a proposal for the Series, please contact:

- David L. Morgan, Series Editor: morgand@pdx.edu
- Helen Salmon, Publisher, Sage: helen.salmon@sagepub.com

S Sage

FOR INFORMATION:

2455 Teller Road
Thousand Oaks, California 91320
Email: order@sagepub.com

1 Oliver's Yard
55 City Road
London EC1Y 1SP
United Kingdom

Unit No 323-333, Third Floor, F-Block
International Trade Tower, Nehru Place
New Delhi – 110 019
India

18 Cross Street #10-10/11/12
China Square Central
Singapore 048423

Copyright © 2025 by Sage.

All rights reserved. Except as permitted by U.S. copyright law, no part of this work may be reproduced or distributed in any form or by any means, or stored in a database or retrieval system, without permission in writing from the publisher.

All third-party trademarks referenced or depicted herein are included solely for the purpose of illustration and are the property of their respective owners. Reference to these trademarks in no way indicates any relationship with, or endorsement by, the trademark owner.

Library of Congress Control Number: 2024028694

ISBN: 978-1-0718-7913-9

This book is printed on acid-free paper.

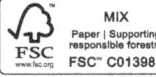

MIX
Paper | Supporting responsible forestry
FSC   FSC™ C013985
www.fsc.org

Printed in the United Kingdom by Henry Ling Limited

Acquisitions Editor: Helen Salmon

Editorial Assistant: Jessica Meyer

Production Editor: Vijayakumar

Copy Editor: Talia Greenberg

Typesetter: TNQ Tech Pvt. Ltd.

Indexer: TNQ Tech Pvt. Ltd.

Cover Designer: Candice Harman

Marketing Manager: Victoria Velasquez

24 25 26 27 28 10 9 8 7 6 5 4 3 2 1

BRIEF CONTENTS

DETAILED CONTENTS

PREFACE

THE INSPIRATION FOR THE BOOK

The idea for this book came while I was creating my own silence, which happened to be while I was sitting and relaxing on the beach. By getting away and cultivating space, I had the idea to create a book to help develop mindful qualitative researchers. This book is the first of its kind, and its purpose is to explore the ways in which mindfulness can enhance the role of the researcher in qualitive inquiry. Many qualitative method texts discuss honing self-reflexivity, developing awareness, or bracketing preexisting knowledge. However, limited texts provide a tool to learn how to exercise reflexivity, cultivate awareness, or identify biases. In addition, few texts provide suggestions to overcome issues that may present themselves in the field. Therefore, this book uses a tangible practice—mindfulness meditation—as a means to train and prepare researchers across disciplines to enter into the field.

OVERVIEW OF THE BOOK

Is this book for you? This book was written with the novice researcher in mind, specifically those navigating a graduate program and being introduced to qualitative methods for the first time. Graduate students at any level may find this book helpful as they learn how to conduct qualitative research methods. However, the skills that can be developed from this book are also helpful for the seasoned researcher who wants fresh eyes and to be reinvigorated about the research process; there is always more room for growth and knowledge. In addition, practitioners who conduct professional research for consumers, brands, or even politicians could benefit from the tools offered in this text.

How should you use this book? This book serves as a training guide to increase our reliability as research instruments and to dive deeper into how mindfulness fits with various aspects of qualitative inquiry. The purpose of this book is to complement other textbooks and reading materials that will be used in the class. For example, during the week(s) that conducting interviews would be covered, Chapter 3 from this book would be read alongside other content to help support what students are learning. Furthermore, if the book is being used in a professional setting, it can be used alongside other training resources that go into greater depth about how to conduct interviews.

Each chapter of this book presents a qualitative method along with a mindfulness practice that stems from the Mindfulness-Based Stress Reduction (MBSR) philosophy and training. The chapter will cover the tenets of that qualitative method, potential issues that may arise in the field, and draw connections to mindfulness by introducing a specific practice that can be learned and incorporated into the research process. Exercises to increase engagement with the topics covered in each chapter and to enhance personal development are also included. At the conclusion of each chapter, directions for a mindfulness practice are provided to deepen self-reflexivity and better attune to the present moment. Key takeaways and points for discussion are also included at the end of each chapter.

The reader is encouraged to complete a writing component, *Mindful Memos*, alongside the practice. The *Mindful Memos* are used to capture how the mind will shift and change over time when using mindfulness. In addition, the *Mindful Memos* serve as short jottings to depict and enhance the researcher's experience with mindfulness. Similar to the memoing process that occurs during data collection and analysis or jottings during participant observation, the *Mindful Memos* assist in describing points of interest. You will find the memos gratifying and illuminating as you witness how your mind transforms over the course of this book.

In addition, the practices are set up to be performed for a week or two before moving on to the next chapter so you can spend time in the practice, which allows for the skills to be experienced and honed before using them prior to data collection or analysis. The time in which one sits in meditation will also increase over the course of the book. This allows you to strengthen your ability to sit in silence over time since it is unrealistic to jump in and complete a 30-minute meditation. It takes time to expand your capacity to sit in intentional silence meditating for a specific period of time, and this book will help you get there.

What will you gain from the book? The culmination of this book is to the incorporate mindfulness practices or interventions into the research process to augment this unique curiosity and heightened awareness to become a mindful qualitative researcher (MQR). The MQR will engage in the practice before entering the field, whether that is a phone or in-person interview, a participant observation, or even conducting a focus group—it just depends on the method of data collection. The practice can also be used alongside data analysis to approach data with openness and nonjudgement. Researchers who engage in this training will be more prepared for the field, establish stronger rapport with participants, collect data that are more trustworthy, and thus make stronger contributions to their fields. Thus, for all the scholars and practitioners who see value in befriending ourselves, thank you for joining me on the journey to becoming mindful qualitative researchers, where we will enrich our findings and—ultimately—our lives.

ACKNOWLEDGMENTS

A few special people need to be recognized for their roles in making this book a reality. To Dr. Joan Rentsch, thank you for offering a mindfulness course while I was pursuing my PhD at the University of Tennessee. The course was life-changing, especially the intentional day of silence, because it ignited my lifelong mindfulness journey. To Dr. Damion Waymer, thank you for being the greatest mentor and encouraging me to pursue this book project. To my dad, thank you for helping me work through my thoughts and ideas over the many miles we hiked together. I am also grateful for the number of times you read and re-read the manuscript, providing thoughtful ideas and suggestions to make the book better. To my mom, thank you for using your incredible artistic talent to inspire and consult on the illustrations for each chapter. It is special to share this project with you in this way. To my husband, thank you for always cheering me on and encouraging me to go after my goals. I am so blessed to have you as my forever partner and friend. And to my son, thank you for being our greatest joy. You truly are as bright as the moon and all the stars combined.

I am also grateful for feedback from the following Sage reviewers during the development of this book:

Theresa Austin, *University of Massachusetts, Amherst*,
Chandra Commuri, *California State University, Bakersfield*,
Linda DeAngelo, *University of Pittsburgh*,
Sandy Guzman-Foster, *University of the Incarnate Word*,
Sally M. Hage, *Springfield College*,
Magdalena Martinez, *University of Nevada, Las Vegas*,
Millicent M. Musyoka, *Lamar University* and
Maaly Yoounis, *University of Northern Colorado*, and
Julie Zadinsky, *Augusta University*.

ABOUT THE AUTHOR

Laura L. Lemon, PhD, is an expert and presenter in the field of public relations who specializes in qualitative methods. Her award-winning research agenda focuses on theory building in internal public relations, with emphasis on internal communication and employee engagement. Her peer-reviewed publications can be found in top journals such as *Journal of Public Relations Research, Public Relations Review, Risk Analysis: An International Journal, Qualitative Market Research: An International Journal*, and *Journal of Communication Management*. Dr. Lemon spent over 7 years as a professional in the private sector assisting organizations with effective public relations initiatives. A passionate and dedicated teacher, Dr. Lemon is a scholar whose research techniques and professional experience support her expertise in the field. She is currently a tenured associate professor at The University of Alabama in the Department of Advertising and Public Relations. Dr. Lemon completed her PhD in communication and information with a public relations focus from the University of Tennessee. She holds a bachelor's degree in communication from Pepperdine University and was conferred a master's in communication from the University of Colorado, Denver.

INTRODUCTION

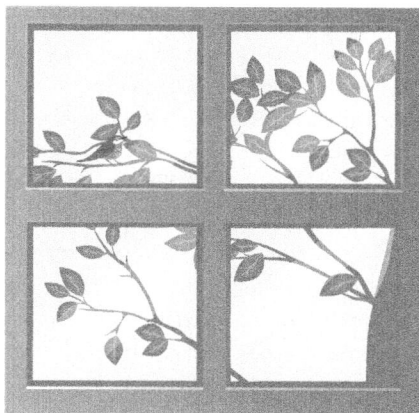

Welcome to exploring the ways in which mindfulness can enhance the role of the researcher in qualitive inquiry. Many qualitative method texts discuss honing self-reflexivity or bracketing preexisting knowledge. However, limited texts provide a tool to exercising reflexivity or identifying biases. In addition, the following chapters provide suggestions to overcoming issues that may present themselves in the field. Therefore, this book will help all qualitative researchers, both novice and experienced, learn how to engage with the present moment and practice mindfulness to enhance our role in qualitive inquiry, adding a pivotal tool to the methodological toolbox.

Ultimately, this book is about creating space. When intentionally generating silence, we are able to cultivate space between thoughts. More often than not, our lives are filled with noise. This is especially true for the research setting, where knowledge, data, and deadlines may overload our minds. Even when we leave the research setting, very rarely are we cultivating quiet in our lives. Time is spent on the phone, using social media, and watching TV, where continuous sounds take up most of the space. Little time is spent cultivating silence because it is often associated with nothingness or a mind dump. However, value exists in cultivating silence. Take, for example, a bird.

The only way a bird will come to an open window is if there is silence. The same philosophy can be applied to our research insights. We cannot create rich insights from data unless we are able to cultivate silence throughout the entire research process.

When we pause and start to recognize the chaos in our environment, silence becomes a source of calm, insight, and focus. Silence helps heighten the senses and increase awareness. When we engage in cultivating intentional silence, we are able to create space. Space leads to an acute attention to thoughts, senses, emotions, sensations, and intensions that may be missed when our mind is filled with noise. The space created from silence leads to further connection with the self. For example, a bowl does not become a bowl until space has been removed for it to fill. A window does not become a window until space has been created to let the light shine in. Similarly, research skills are honed and enhanced when space is created in the mind. A few moments of silence can grow and deepen contemplation, help us turn inward, and focus our attention, which ultimately creates more space in our mind. Silence creates room for us to deepen our connection to ourselves and those around us, which enhances our research abilities. Let us take a deeper dive into better understanding mindfulness.

WHAT IS MINDFULNESS?

Defining Mindfulness. In the most basic explanation, mindfulness is an awareness that occurs from paying attention on purpose. Kabat-Zinn (2003) defined mindfulness as "an awareness that emerges through paying attention on purpose, in the present moment, and practicing non-judgment of the experience throughout each moment" (p. 145). Mindfulness is characterized by a nonjudgmental awareness that creates a special kind of attention rooted in openness and curiosity. When we exercise this level of attention, the result is a profound acceptance of *all* experiences, both internal and external (Chiesa & Serretti, 2009). Through the practice of meditation, the focus is on developing our ability to exercise a nonjudgmental awareness and welcoming of all experiences (Kabat-Zinn, 2003). Over time, when we exercise this special kind of attention we begin to avoid acting impulsively and instead operate from a thoughtful and intentional place (Chiesa & Serretti, 2009).

The Systemic Approach. Beyond honing the skill to pay attention on purpose, mindfulness occurs through body awareness, where emotions are regulated to the extent that certain emotional responses are avoided, and perspectives of the self adjust, which cultivates a higher level of self-acceptance (Hozel et al., 2011). Shapiro and Schwartz (2000) provided the Intentional Systemic Mindfulness (ISM) model, which serves as the theoretical construct to elucidate the interrelatedness of self-regulation, attitude, and the intention that occurs when practicing mindfulness. The mindfulness experience does not follow a linear process; rather, it encompasses the constant ebb and flow of expanding and redefining the initial intention behind the practice. Mindfulness is cultivated through the interconnectedness between the experiences of self-regulation, attitude, and intention. Specifically, Shapiro and Schwartz (2002) explained that self-regulation, or the role of attention, is the process through which the system maintains the stability to function while incorporating flexibility and the capacity for change in new situations. When we function with flexibility, the capacity for change leads to self-regulation. The end result is order and health across the entire system or person.

In using this systemic perspective, self-regulation recognizes the interrelatedness of all things. This leads to the intention of accepting and healing each piece of the system, while simultaneously restoring the larger whole. To heal the system, the individual must employ an attitude grounded in the mindfulness qualities to enable self-regulation (Shapiro & Schwartz, 2002). Mindfulness qualities include letting go, openness, patience, acceptance, nonstriving, trust, and nonjudgment. These attitudes lead to the development of regulated emotional responses like loving-kindness, gratitude, empathy, generosity, and gentleness. The ISM approach illustrates that the mindfulness practice is more than simply paying attention; what is most important is the intention behind the attention regulation that results from mindful practices.

Mindfulness-Based Stress Reduction (MBSR)

To develop mindfulness, one must participate in programs like Mindfulness-Based Stress Reduction, which systematically uses mindful attention to cultivate aspects of the mind and heart (Kabat-Zinn, 2003). The MBSR program helps people develop mindfulness, by making one radically aware of the present moment, accepting the moment as it is without becoming caught up in the emotions and thoughts that may arise within the experience (Shapiro, Astin, Bishop, & Cordova, 2005). The MBSR program teaches three different practices: the body scan, which includes a slow-moving attention across the body from head to feet, concentrating on any sensation or feeling that may occur in the body; sitting meditation, where the focus is on the breath and a state of nonjudgmental awareness as thoughts and distractions continually arise in the mind and in the space; and a Hatha yoga practice, which incorporates simple stretches and breathing exercises (Chiesa & Serretti, 2009).

Aligning with the ISM approach, I believe mindfulness is more than a yoga or meditation practice. Mindfulness is about a profound acceptance, where all states of mind are embraced, without striving for or favoring one state of mind over the other and embracing whatever is occurring in the present moment because it is already happening (Kabat-Zinn, 2005). The mindfulness practice is a way of being. It is about exercising an intention to pay attention on purpose, relying on the attitudes that underpin mindfulness, and simply experiencing the present moment just as it is.

THE QUALITATIVE RESEARCHER

When inquiry is rooted in the participants' experiences, where those experiences develop insights, the researcher is conducting qualitative research. Qualitative researchers focus on how people experience their own natural environment and how they give meaning to that experience (Chesebro & Borisoff, 2007). Inquiries from a qualitative tradition are defined by four main characteristics (Merriam & Tisdell, 2016). First, data collection is about focusing on and understanding meaning from the participants' lived experience. Second, the process is inductive, where the data gathered is used to build concepts, theories, hypotheses. Third, the findings include rich descriptions, where words are used for data collection instead of numbers. The goal is to not quantify but to explain. The fourth, and most important for this text, is that the researcher is the primary instrument.

There are advantages to the researcher being the instrument, such as processing information immediately and asking participants to clarify information while engaging in data collection. However, issues do arise when the researcher is the instrument. Specifically, all researchers arrive with personal biases, existing information, and preconceived notions about the research setting. While these are human nature, since our previous experiences shape who we are, working to deal with personal biases and preexisting knowledge is an important process for any qualitative researcher. This highly personal process helps ensure trustworthiness throughout the entire research investigation.

To be a proficient qualitative researcher, we must participate in training. Training can come in the form of traditional coursework, special conference sessions, or reading texts focused on methods. While engaging with these various trainings, the researcher can become more reliable (Merriam & Tisdell, 2016). Since the researcher is both the data collection and data analysis instrument, training to hone the skills that reinforce this experience is necessary. Specifically, how can a researcher train to be more present, welcome ambiguity, exercise curiosity, increase awareness, and practice empathy to respond accordingly to whatever may occur in the research setting? The answer is to develop a research-based mindfulness practice, which is the focus for this book.

When qualitative researchers incorporate mindfulness, we are motivated by acute curiosity and open-mindedness about whatever the research setting and the participant(s) bring up. In addition, we remain engaged and present in the research process despite preexisting knowledge, thoughts, and habits that may detract from the present moment (Stetler, 2010). Such practice would help the bricoleur augment crystallization, which "requires patience and zen-like contemplation" (Stewart, Gapp, & Harwood, 2017, p. 13). We would also exercise a deep empathy while interacting and sharing the research setting with participants. The next section further explicates the connection between a mindfulness practice and the qualitative researcher.

THE MINDFUL QUALITATIVE RESEARCHER

Life as a researcher is often characterized by strict deadlines and information overload, where decisions are pragmatically made to meet job requirements and goals. However, to value every step of the research process, qualitative researchers must prioritize and carve out thinking time to safeguard thought processes (Keegan, 2012). The only way to do this is to turn off the technology, explore nature, and invite in all aspects of the human experience, which leads to a commitment to exist and live in the present moment. This way of life has great potential to make a difference in our lives, our participants' lives, and the research community as a whole (Lemon, 2017). We can then be liberated from limiting thoughts to refine our minds and our potential for seeing and knowing (Kabat-Zinn, 2005). Mindfulness is an invitation to get to know ourselves better through each present moment (2005).

At the foundation, mindfulness is rooted in rich inquiry and the finesse of insights (Kabat-Zinn, 2005), which means a natural connection exists between the qualitative researcher and mindfulness. As mentioned previously, qualitative research is focused on locating the researcher *inside* the participants' world, where the goal of data collection is to capture the participants' point of view and lived experience (Denzin & Lincoln, 2013). Although not openly discussed in extant literature (e.g., Brummans, 2014), qualitative researchers could benefit from incorporating mindfulness into data collection and analysis since the practice is about being in the present moment and paying attention on purpose. Most importantly, this skill would eradicate the researcher moving through the research setting on autopilot with an undisciplined mind, which could result in the researcher's mind becoming an unreliable tool (Hart et al., 2013). In the end, you will transition into being a mindful qualitative researcher.

The Benefits. From a broad perspective, the mindfulness practice offers three advantages. First, mindfulness can assist with the researcher and participant relationship. The researcher and participant are fused into a single reality, where knowledge emerges from this unique exchange (Lincoln, Lynham, & Guba, 2013); ultimately, the researcher and the participant are inextricably connected (Lincoln & Guba, 1985). The mindfulness practice strengthens this intentional relationship between the researcher and the participant and enhances the researcher's curiosity, openness, and awareness that facilitate the research process. Cultivating awareness through mindfulness removes the dualistic relationship of researcher versus participant and encourages an intentional relationship where both are engaging in the co-creation of data, which is one of the unique strengths of qualitative research (Brummans, 2014).

Second, mindfulness can be used to support the notion of the emergent research design and can help researchers exercise flexibility while in the research setting (Lemon, 2017). The mindfulness practice helps the researcher embrace the idea that the phenomenon can and should emerge on its own without controlling the process, where the goal is to adopt and welcome an emergent design. The concept of the emergent design encourages the researcher to navigate whatever presents itself in the field and to let things simply occur, instead of forcing and imposing predetermined assumptions and meanings onto the research setting. A skilled qualitative researcher is competent in dealing with ambiguity and carefully observing in the midst of uncertainty (Merriam & Tisdell, 2016). Yin (2014) offered that a skilled researcher will adapt to the research setting and avoid biases when possible. Mindfulness entails a unique openness to all events or situations because the practice reminds us that everyday life is constantly changing; this prevents the predetermination.

Third, mindfulness can help hone self-reflexivity. Important note: Mindfulness and self-reflexivity are not one and the same; rather, mindfulness can enrich our abilities to exercise reflexivity. Self-reflexivity is about researchers recognizing their position within the participants' world (Merriam & Tisdell, 2016). In employing self-reflexivity, the researcher explains existing biases, knowledge, and assumptions regarding the research investigation. The mindfulness practice is actually greater than self-reflexivity because the practice encourages the practitioner to become extremely aware of the *full* experience, which is occurring in the present moment, moving beyond the bank of preexisting knowledge. This would lead researchers who practice mindfulness to recognize the many ways in which we often edit our experiences in addition to the biases and assumptions. When experiences are edited, we misrepresent the present moment by relying on routine and habitual behaviors that estrange our current experience (Kabat-Zinn, 2005). Incorporating mindfulness as a tool for qualitative researchers could potentially lessen habitual thought processes, providing an opportunity to attend to more subtle thoughts that would ordinarily be ignored (Buttle, 2013). The end result is potentially more nuanced and richer findings from data collection and analysis.

LEARNING HOW TO MINDFULLY MEMO

Before concluding, let's discuss a unique component of each chapter in this book: the *Mindful Memos*. *Mindful Memos* are a journaling aspect that encourage a deeper connection to the physical meditation practices in this book. The purpose of the *Mindful Memos* is to see how your mind shifts and changes over the course of each 2-week practice. These changes may be very subtle, so without the memos, any nuance of the experiences may be missed.

After learning a new meditation practice, you will be asked to memo about your experiences. The following questions can be used to guide what you write in the *Mindful Memos*. But remember these questions are just a guide to get you started. I encourage you to explore other questions that fit best with your experience.

- How did you feel before the meditation, throughout, and then after?

- What unique physical sensations did you have throughout the meditation?

- Did you experience any physical pain? Where did you experience that pain?

- Was your mind drawn to the same thought or previous experience over and over? What was that thought?

- Did you find yourself planning, making lists, or ruminating about the past?

- What changes are you seeing in your thought processes because of your new meditation practice?

- Anything unique, interesting, or important stand out to you regarding your experience?

As mentioned, these are questions to initiate what you might capture in the *Mindful Memos*. Feel free to write just a few notes or more, depending on what you feel most comfortable with at the time. However, the *Mindful Memos* should be captured after each meditation practice. The *Mindful Memos* should also be reviewed following the 2-week practice. In doing so, the change that is fundamental to having a consistent meditation practice will be witnessed.

CONCLUSION

This chapter provided an overview of the book in addition to the mindfulness practice, setting the stage for what to expect in the following pages. Connections were made between mindfulness and qualitative research to demonstrate how this practice can benefit researchers at various stages in their careers.

KEY TAKEAWAYS

- Ultimately, this book is about creating space to enhance and improve qualitative research. When intentionally generating silence, we cultivate space between thoughts. Silence creates room for us to deepen our connection to ourselves and those around us, which enhances our research abilities.

- Mindfulness is an awareness that occurs from paying attention on purpose. When qualitative researchers incorporate mindfulness, we are motivated by acute curiosity and open-mindedness about whatever the research setting and the participant(s) bring up.

- This book serves as a training guide to increase our reliability as research instruments and to dive deeper into how mindfulness fits with various aspects of qualitative inquiry. Each chapter of this book presents a qualitative method along with a mindfulness practice that stems from the MBSR philosophy and training.

REFLECTION QUESTIONS

- Have you heard of "mindfulness" prior to reading this chapter? What are your initial impressions of mindfulness?

- What concerns do you have about pursuing a mindfulness practice?

- What barriers might you face while pursuing the mindfulness practices presented in this book? How might you overcome those barriers?

- What do you think about the *Mindful Memos*? How will you incorporate this component into your meditation practice?

REFERENCES AND FURTHER READING

Brummans, B. H. J. M. (2014). Pathways to mindful qualitative organizational communication research. *Management Communication Quarterly, 28*, 440–447.

Buttle, H. (2013). More than the sum of my parts: A cognitive psychologist reflects on mindfulness/meditation experience. *Reflective Practice: International and Multidisciplinary Perspectives, 14*, 766–773.

Chesebro, J. W., & Borisoff, D. J. (2007). What makes qualitative research qualitative? *Qualitative Research Reports in Communication, 8*(1), 3–14.

Chiesa, A., & Serretti, A. (2009). Mindfulness-based stress reduction for stress management in healthy people: A review of literature and meta-analysis. *The Journal of Alternative and Complementary Medicine, 15*, 593–600.

Denzin, N. K., & Lincoln, Y. S. (2013). The discipline and practice of qualitative research. In *The landscape of qualitative research* (4th ed.). Sage.

Hart, R., Ivtzan, I., & Hart, D. (2013). Mind the gap in mindfulness research: A comparative account of the leading schools of thought. *Review of General Psychology, 17*, 453–466.

Hozel, B. K., Lazar, S. W., Gard, T., Schuman-Olivier, Z., Vago, D. R., & Ott, U. (2011). How does mindfulness meditation work? Proposing mechanisms of action from a conceptual and neural perspective. *Perspectives of Psychological Science, 6*, 537–559.

Kabat-Zinn, J. (2003). Mindfulness-based interventions in context: Past, present, and future. *Clinical Psychology: Science and Practice, 10*, 144–156.

Kabat-Zinn, J. (2005). Meditation—It's not what you think. *Mindfulness, 6*, 393–395.

Keegan, S. (2012). Digital technologies are re-shaping our brains. *Qualitative Market Research: An International Journal, 15*, 328–346.

Lemon, L. (2017). Applying a mindfulness practice to qualitative data collection. *The Qualitative Report, 22*(12), 3305–3313.

Lincoln, Y. S., & Guba, E. G. (1985). *Naturalistic inquiry.* Sage.

Lincoln, Y. S., Lynham, S. A., & Guba, E. G. (2013). Paradigmatic controversies, contradictions, and emerging confluences, revisited. In *The landscape of qualitative research* (4th ed.). Sage.

Merriam, S. B., & Tisdell, E. J. (2016). *Qualitative research: A guide to design and implementation* (4th ed.). Jossey-Bass.

Shapiro, S. L., Astin, J. A., Bishop, S. R., & Cordova, M. (2005). Mindfulness-based stress reduction for health care professionals: Results from randomized trial. *International Journal of Stress Management, 12,* 164–176.

Shapiro, S. L., & Schwartz, G. E. (2000). The role of intention in self-regulation: Toward intentional systemic mindfulness. In *Handbook of Self-Regulation,* 253–273. Academic Press.

Stelter, R. (2010). Experience-based, body-anchored qualitative research interviewing. *Qualitative Health Research, 20,* 859–867.

Stewart, H., Gapp, R., & Harwood, I. (2017). Exploring the alchemy of qualitative management research: Seeking trustworthiness, credibility and rigor through crystallization. *The Qualitative Report, 22*(1), 1–19.

Yin, R. K. (2014). *Case study research: Design and methods* (5th ed.). Sage.

2 EXPLORING THE SELF BY LEARNING TO LISTEN

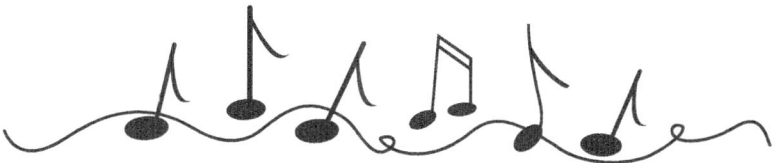

This chapter, Exploring the Self by Learning to Listen, focuses on researchers' experiences with the self and how they may overcome personal perceived obstacles such as perfectionism and confidence during the research process. By introducing a meditation that focuses on sound, the researcher learns how to welcome in the present moment instead of getting carried away with ruminating thoughts of future predictions or previous experiences. This chapter will also help readers investigate the "researcher self" by giving them the chance to consider their own ontology and epistemology. The chapter ends with a conclusion, key takeaways, and reflection questions. A space for the *Mindful Memos* is included along with a summary of the practice.

EXPLORING THE "RESEARCHER SELF"

Who you are and what you believe matters when you show up to the research setting. Awareness of your past experiences and the knowledge you have gained makes a difference in how you interact with participants through data collection and the insights garnered through data analysis. It is reasonable to have experiences and knowledge that shape the way you think, but awareness of it is key.

Let me share a story to illustrate. I had a former student who was studying to earn his master's degree. I was serving on his thesis committee as the member who would oversee his method of choice. He was interested in conducting interviews with members of the debate community to capture how the COVID-19 pandemic changed the practice of debate by moving it to an online format. It was an insightful idea for a study, especially since this is the first time this community experienced major changes. This was also an ideal topic for him because he was passionate about it—great research ideas often come from topics with which we are ardent. He spent years in the debate community, initially as an undergraduate student debater and later, a debate coach and judge.

Given his proximity to and previous experience with the debate community, I encouraged him to include a statement of researcher reflexivity into the proposal. This was an opportunity for him to reflect on his connection to the topic and how that might impact data collection and analysis. A statement of researcher positionality or reflexivity is where the investigator explores in writing the impact of the research process on the self as well as the influence of the researcher on the research process (Probst & Berenson, 2014). Specifically, Probst and Berenson (2014) defined reflexivity as "awareness of the influence the researcher has on what is being studied and, simultaneously, of how the research process affects the researcher. It is both a state of mind and a set of actions" (p. 64).

At his defense, he discussed the theories he connected with most as his researcher reflexivity instead of his experience with the debate community. It took some time in our discussion for him to realize what we (the committee) meant by investigating his own experiences and knowledge and how both will inform his research process. For example, his research questions were written with value-laden language that reflected his potential biases. We brought this to his attention as well as other elements of the proposal that mirrored his experiences. Therefore, for his revised proposal, we challenged him to start with reflexivity so that he could identify how his experiences may inform the project and how he plans to position himself within that understanding and expertise. The committee and I assured him that in spending time unveiling his insider perspective, he would enrich and strengthen his final project.

The Role of Ontology and Epistemology. The first step in assessing one's position within research is to understand how ontology and epistemology impact the research process. Ontology is defined as the worldview and assumptions or view of reality from which researchers operate in their quest for original knowledge (Schwandt, 2007). "An ontological view conceives of or apprehends the world from a specific standpoint" (Arneson, 2009a, p. 696). What topics scholars choose to study and how they elucidate the findings of their research mirror the assumptions they make about the world around them (Arneson, 2009a). Distinctive ontologies are going to result in alternative understandings, which lead to differences in conceptualizing and theorizing about the topic under investigation (Arneson, 2009a). For a full description of all the different ontologies and to learn more about the different ontological positions, see Merriam and Tisdell (2016).

Epistemology deals with exploring what is knowledge and the understanding of how knowledge is generated (Lincoln, Lynham, & Guba, 2013). This philosophical perspective assesses "the nature, scope, and limits of human knowledge" (Arneson, 2009b, p. 351). It is the science of knowing (Babbie, 2013), and seeks to uncover the relationship between the researcher and the known (Lindlof & Taylor, 2011). In other words, epistemological assumptions center around knowledge generation and "how we come to know what we think we know" (Arneson, 2009b, p. 350). For a full synopsis of epistemological stances, I encourage you to pursue additional reading to uncover your epistemological alignment (see Tracy, 2020).

My Researcher Positionality Statement. You will be encouraged to reflect on your alignment and stances as a researcher here shortly. But before you do, I think it is beneficial to see an example. Below is my researcher positionality statement.

I position myself as a qualitative researcher who aligns with the interpretivist ontology and epistemology. From this perspective, I understand that the knowledge of social reality arises from the essential interconnection that exists between the researcher and participants. The researcher and participants that are *invited* to be in the study are connected in such a way that who they are and how they view and understand the world are fundamental to how they process and make meaning of themselves, others, and the world around them (Guba & Lincoln, 1994).

As an interpretive scholar, I understand that methodological instruments are not used in a void, but rather we, the researchers, are the instruments to guide the methods (cf. Lindlof & Taylor, 2011). Interpretivist scholars cannot separate who we are and what we know from the research experiences, since our ontology and epistemology are cultivated by and supported throughout our lived experiences. The result is knowledge claims that reflect both the experiences of the researcher and the participants. Through rigorous data analysis, the lived experiences of the participants are brought to the forefront to be examined and understood.

In addition to being an interpretive qualitative researcher, I am also a communication scholar. Specifically, I study internal communication and employee engagement under the umbrella of public relations. My scholarship centers on understanding the employees' lived experience, so that organizations can develop meaningful internal communication that supports a healthy and productive work environment. I provide theoretical and practical implications to facilitate and promote the fundamental understanding that employees are not a means to an end, but instead are human beings with intrinsic value. Given my involvement and awareness with this subject matter, I arrive at all research settings with my own perceptions and experiences. Although this knowledge cannot be removed or ignored, it can be acknowledged and therefore curbed during the different stages of a research study to ensure I stay open to the participants' experiences and not be induced by my own.

Taking the Researcher Positionality One Step Further. As discussed above, my ontology and epistemology inform the way in which I view knowledge generation and the research process. Furthermore, I wrote this book from an interpretivist vantage point because this is the way in which I see the world. The examples used in this book also reflect the field of communication since it's my research and teaching background. However, this doesn't mean that a critical scholar or a post-positivist scholar cannot use the tools presented in this book; in fact, I encourage them. Similarly, people from different disciplines will also have much to gain from the narratives and skills presented in this book. I simply share this information to articulate and clarify to the readers my point of view in the following text. In doing so, readers are clear as to how my values and expectations influenced the words written in the book. Clarity in one's research position matters, and we should all be striving to inform readers of our assumptions, dispositions, and experiences regarding the research process.

As you pursue your own research endeavors, I encourage you to include a researcher positionality statement in the method section of your manuscripts. Many journals expect this information to be included in submissions. From my own publishing experience, I have had editors request my researcher positionality statement be integrated in the final version of a manuscript. I also suggest to scholars whose work I am reviewing to incorporate this information. By including a statement that articulates who we are as researchers, readers can learn about our particular values and expectations and how those guided the research process and influenced the insights of the study (Maxwell, 2013).

GIVE THE RESEARCHER POSITIONALITY STATEMENT A TRY!

Now, it is your turn to write your position as a researcher. First, consider your research interests. What discipline does you research fall under? Why are you interested in studying certain topics? What contributions do you hope to make with your research? Second, contemplate your ontology and epistemology. Explore extra reading, since this chapter covered the basic definition of both. How would you describe your ontology and epistemology? How will these beliefs impact you and your participants' experience? I encourage you to write freely while considering these questions—not focusing on getting it right, but instead creating your narrative on paper so you can begin to reflect on your position.

RESEARCHER ROADBLOCKS AND LISTENING IN THE PRESENT MOMENT TO WORK THROUGH THEM

As mentioned, our knowledge and experiences bolster who we are when we show up to the researcher setting. However, we might have personal roadblocks that stifle our abilities as researchers. Those might include a lack of confidence when learning a new method and perfectionism. Mindfulness practices can be a useful tool to overcome these limitations. Specifically, the listening meditation can help bring us back to the present moment, and out of our own heads. In other words, many of our limitations are perceived and not a true depiction of reality. This means we must overcome the mental narratives we tell ourselves about what we can and cannot do. Some of those narratives have been with us for most of our lives because of the experiences we have had, what we have learned, or the messages communicated to us. These narratives are thoughts, and thoughts do not define who we are. Thoughts are simply thoughts—nothing more, nothing less.

However, the thoughts we have about our confidence in the research setting—whether we *should* be conducting this type of research, or only submitting a project if it is perfect—can limit our ability to move forward and collect quality data that make a difference in our respective fields either in practice or through theory development. One solution to navigating these emotions and experiences is to focus on the present moment by using sound.

Sounds are all around us and can help tether us to the present moment. What this means is that when your mind begins to drift into a negative or limiting thought about your abilities or experiences, you can bring yourself out of that thought by focusing on the sounds around you. Sometimes, we can get hung up on these thoughts, but sounds can be the tool out of the trance. Let's dive into how these might play out in the research setting and how the listening meditation can assist with navigating these experiences.

Limited Confidence. As with all things that are new, we may not have the confidence to pursue it. As novices in the research arena, like with employing a new method of data collection, we might be intimidated to give it a try. For example, if you are an experienced qualitative researcher who has relied on interviews and focus groups for data collection, when embarking on participant observations, you may have some reservations. Or maybe you are a quantitative researcher who has never conducted an interview; you may lack the confidence you tend to have when administering a survey. This lack of confidence may lead some academics and researchers to experience imposter syndrome. Imposter syndrome is defined as "doubting your abilities and feeling like a fraud at work" (Tulshyan & Burey, 2021, p. 1). This is a natural response to being new at something, which means one may lack confidence in their abilities.

Let me illustrate with an example, which shows that even the most experienced scholars sometimes run into confidence issues. I have been working on a grant-funded project with colleagues in my department. We are conducting interviews with professionals in our fields regarding their opinions on disinformation. I am the only qualitative scholar on the team, and the other three researchers are experts in quantitative methods. Prior to collecting data, I led a brief training session on how to conduct interviews. I also encouraged my team to practice listening to sounds in the present moment anytime they started to doubt their abilities. This prompted them to not get swept away in limiting thought processes and brought them back to the present moment so they could focus on the task at hand: having great conversations with professionals in our field.

Perfectionism. Another individual limitation a researcher may face is perfectionism. Social work scholar and *New York Times* best-selling author Brené Brown has researched the confines and implications of perfectionism. Specifically, perfectionism "can be exhausting because hustling is exhausting. It's a never-ending performance" (Brown, 2012, p. 133). It can also be crushing to our creativity (Brown, 2012). Therefore, perfectionism has the potential to restrict the researcher throughout various places in the research process.

From my experience, students can often be hindered by the need to be perfect. The unrealistic expectations students place on themselves impact their willingness to learn by taking risks. These risks may mean that the end grade does not reflect their initial hopes of earning top marks. However, in making mistakes and accepting imperfections, learning ensues, and knowledge is gained.

I have one previous student who stands out in my mind that we could all emulate since she was not stifled by perfectionism. She was willing to take risks in the classroom in ways I have never seen from a student. Most of the time, graduate and undergraduate students are most concerned about their grade and make calculated steps to ensure they get the best grade possible. Very rarely do students seek to learn simply for the experience of learning; most students are interested in learning to receive a grade. However, this particular student was different. She was willing to take risks in learning a new method, attempting a different way of writing, and accepted that since it was new, she may not be great at it the first time. Her willingness to hit a few bumps in the beginning paid off generously as she advanced quicker than some of her peers in the class simply because she was willing to take risks and was not stifled by perfectionism.

We may not all have the skills or experiences that support the willingness to take risks and be imperfect. However, a listening meditation can be one tool to help ground us in the present moment when our minds try to take us down the path of thinking we need to be perfect. Perfectionism tells us that we can't do good enough, or that what we have done isn't good enough—but nothing is truly perfect, which is hard to believe when we spend so much time online in a curated world. By focusing on listening to sounds in the present moment when our minds start to trail off with thoughts and desires for a perfect research study or a perfect paper, we can stop the ruminating so that we can move forward. Without this tool, we will become exhausted and unproductive by the overpowering desire to always be perfect. The next section offers a step-by-step approach to learn how to listen for sounds to forget any preconceived desire for control and perfectionism.

THE PRACTICE: LISTENING TO SOUNDS MEDITATION

Meditation is a practice, which means it takes some time to learn how to sit in silence. However, even after years of practice, some days can be harder than others to sit and focus on being present in the moment. This can be humbling, and it helps encourage us to always return to the practice because we never "conquer" meditation.

The following practice is going to introduce you to meditation by first focusing on your breath and then focusing on sound. This will be an "easier" meditation and a great place to start if you have never meditated before. Again, using sound can help bring us into the present moment so we can get out of our minds and ruminating thoughts. Let us begin.

You will want to begin this meditation by finding a quiet place to sit. Be sure you are comfortable so you can sit for 10 minutes in the same place without distractions. We will be building up the time we spend meditating over the course of this book—so let's start with an achievable amount of time and set a timer for 10 minutes. Your sitting position should be active and alert yet relaxed at the same time. Remember, this is most likely your first time meditating, so be sure to be compassionate and understanding with yourself if you find the practice difficult. Even if you find it hard, you will try again tomorrow. The most experienced practitioners have hard days too, so it is not a big deal if you find your mind all over the place.

Start by sitting in a comfortable position with a straight back. Take a deep breath and audibly exhale. Close your eyes. Rest your hands gently in your lap or on your knees. Relax your neck and shoulders. Relax the muscles in your face. Take another deep, audible breath and feel your body begin to relax.

As you settle into this moment, begin focusing on your breath. Hear yourself breath in and then breath out. Focus on the quiet moment that happens at the end of every exhale and at the beginning of every inhale. You will see there is a gentle pause at the beginning and end of every exhale.

To help calm the mind, focus on counting to 10. At the end of one cycle of breath, where you complete one inhale and then one exhale, count one. Inhale deeply and exhale, then count two. Inhale and exhale, then count three. Continue in this way until you reach 10.

Now, let us transition the practice to listening to sounds. Begin by noticing in this moment the sounds in the room. What do you hear? Do you hear a sound in your immediate space? Are you able to hear sounds that are far away? As you focus on sounds, be sure not to get lost in thinking about the sounds or focusing on what is making the sound or labeling the sound. Just rest in the experience of listening, without judging or identifying the sound; sit with the raw vibrations that are the essence of hearing sounds.

Be open and explore the sounds that you could not hear at the beginning of the meditation. Sounds will come and go throughout the meditation. You might hear sounds from the body, from the room you are in, or from nature outside. There might also be times when there are no sounds; in this case, focus on the silence. You have nothing to do, nothing to fix or change about this moment, but accept it exactly as it is.

In terms of awareness, know that all sounds are equal. Yet you might gravitate toward certain sounds, liking some and disliking others. See if it is possible to rest in awareness of hearing without quantifying the sounds, letting go of the stories you might have about these particular sounds. Also know that you might be aware of thoughts, feelings, and body sensations. This is quite natural. But keep bringing your attention back to simply hearing.

Once the timer goes off, begin to slowly move your body, and open your eyes to bring yourself back into the room. Notice how you feel? How does your body feel? How does your mind feel? How can you take this sharp, focused attention into the rest of your day? Take a few minutes to pay attention to the experience of focusing your mind on the present moment for a period of time using sound. Record your thoughts, feelings, and sensations about the experience in your *Mindful Memos*.

The listening to sounds meditation will be your practice for the next 2 weeks. Dedicate 10 minutes each day to this meditation. Throughout the next 2 weeks of practice and memoing you will begin to see small changes. Be sure to come to the practice every day with an open mind no matter what your experience was like the previous day or what type of experience you hope to have that day. To see how you change and evolve over time, come to the practice every day with an open mind. It is important to complete the *Mindful Memos* at the end of each meditation so the small changes can be captured. The nuance will be missed without the memos. This practice sets the foundation for others you will encounter in the upcoming chapters.

CONCLUSION

This chapter began by discussing the researcher self, including brief definitions of ontology and epistemology. A researcher positionality statement section was included, which encourages the development of an individual statement. Limitations of the researcher's thoughts were also discussed, and the listening to sounds meditation was introduced as a way to navigate the desire for control and perfectionism. The steps to the listening to sounds meditation were included, which is the meditation that should be practiced over the next 2 weeks. This mindfulness practice will give researchers an introduction to meditation, providing them a useful exercise to practice tuning into the present moment so that limiting beliefs are left behind and forgotten.

KEY TAKEAWAYS

- Who you are and what you believe matter when you show up to the research setting. Awareness of your past experiences and the knowledge you have gained make a difference in how you interact with participants through data collection and the insights garnered through data analysis.

- The first step in assessing one's position within research is to understand how ontology and epistemology impact the research process.

- Researchers are encouraged to include a positionality statement in the method section of future manuscripts.

- We might have personal roadblocks that stifle our abilities as researchers. Those might include a lack of confidence when learning a new method and perfectionism.

- The listening to sounds meditation can be one tool to help ground us in the present moment when our minds try to take us down the path of believing we cannot do something or striving for perfectionism.

REFLECTION QUESTIONS

- Based on what you have learned, what is your ontological stance? Where do you align in terms of your epistemology? How do you think these vantage points will inform your research process?

- What concerns do you have about conducting research? What components of the research process excite you?

- How might your previous experiences inform the research topics you are interested in studying?

- Have you written a researcher reflexivity or positionality statement? If so, what was that experience like for you? If not, how do you feel about capturing your experience and knowledge on paper?

THE 2-WEEK PRACTICE: LISTENING TO SOUNDS MEDITATION

The listening to sounds meditation will be your meditation practice for the next 2 weeks. Dedicate time each day to the listening to sounds meditation to see how you are learning to hone your focus and access the present moment through sound. At the end of each daily meditation, complete a mindful memo that captures your experience. The memos are key to capturing the nuance of how your practice will shift and change over time. Be prepared to welcome whatever arises during your first few meditations. Most importantly, be patient and open with your experience as you learn a new skill.

Mindful Memos

REFERENCES

Arneson, P. (2009a). Ontology. In S. W. Littlejohn & K. A. Foss (Eds.), *Encyclopedia of communication theory* (Volume 2; pp. 695–698). Sage.

Arneson, P. (2009b). Epistemology. In S. W. Littlejohn & K. A. Foss (Eds.), *Encyclopedia of communication theory* (Volume 1; pp. 349–352). Sage.

Babbie, E. (2013). *The practice of social research* (13th ed.). Wadsworth.

Brown, B. (2012). *Daring greatly: How the courage to be vulnerable transforms the way we live, love, parent, and lead.* Gotham Books.

Guba, E. G., & Lincoln, Y. S. (1994). Competing paradigms in qualitative research. In N. K. Denzin & Y. S. Lincoln (Eds.), *Handbook of qualitative research.* Sage.

Lincoln, Y. S., Lynham, S. A., & Guba, E. G. (2013). Paradigmatic controversies, contradictions, and emerging confluences, revisited. In *The landscape of qualitative research* (4th ed.). Sage.

Lindlof, T. R., & Taylor, B. C. (2011). *Qualitative communication research methods* (3rd ed.). Sage.

Maxwell, J. A. (2013). *Qualitative research design: An interactive approach* (3rd ed.). Sage.

Probst, B., & Berenson, L. (2014). The double arrow: How qualitative social work researchers use reflexivity. *Qualitative Social Work, 13*(6), 813–827.

Schwandt, T. A. (2007). *The SAGE dictionary of qualitative inquiry* (3rd ed.). Sage.

Tracy, S. J. (2020). *Qualitative research methods: Collecting evidence, crafting analysis, communicating impact* (2nd ed.). Wiley-Blackwell.

Tulshyan, R., & Burey, J.-A. (2021). Stop telling women they have imposter syndrome. *Harvard Business Review.* Retrieved on July 7, 2022, at https://hbr.org/2021/02/stop-telling-women-they-have-imposter-syndrome

3 INTERVIEWING WITH A BEGINNER'S MIND

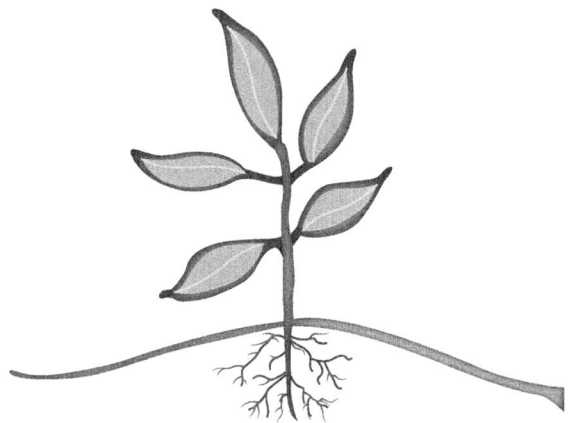

The third chapter, Interviewing With a Beginner's Mind, begins with an overview of the beginner's mind. The interview as a data collection tool is then discussed, followed by probable issues one may face while interviewing. The beginner's mind is integrated throughout the challenges section, which is a tool for the researcher to use to potentially tackle some of the issues one may face in the field. The body scan practice is then introduced, which is a meditation practice that helps develop the beginner's mind. The chapter ends with a space for the *Mindful Memos* to capture what is learned from nurturing the beginner's mind.

A BEGINNER'S MIND

A beginner's mind is about approaching life with an attitude of openness. This mindset allows us to see the world through fresh eyes and with open ears. To do so, we must put away our existing beliefs to free ourselves from any limiting preconceptions and biases. As researchers, most of us have goals to become experts in our fields. This is natural, since we want to be viewed as someone who is informed and knowledgeable, and it feels good when we *think* we have all of the answers. Ironically, having all the answers doesn't allow for new understanding and insights to come to fruition. The beginner's mind allows us to reset our thought processes and start anew to welcome in new insights and information, which is useful while conducting interviews.

A beginner's mind allows the researcher to cultivate a new level of awareness by seeing the research process like it's the first time, even though it may be the hundredth time. It allows both the experienced and novice researchers to interview study participants with open eyes and ears. When we bring a beginner's mind to the research process, we stop being limited by our beliefs about others, and instead see them as they really are: unique and interesting. Thus, we stop being limited by our beliefs about ourselves and others. Bringing this kind of attention to the table ensures people feel seen, which is especially important in the research setting. In doing so, we avoid getting trapped in prior assumptions, perceptions, or knowledge. When we get unstuck about our opinions, beliefs, ideas, and outcomes and replace them with a fresh openness, we welcome in tremendous possibilities. These possibilities turn into rich details and insights that are fundamental to qualitative research. If our mind is full, there is no opportunity to add additional information and knowledge. We are unable to observe things without judgment, and we miss the chance to see the possibilities of what could be in terms of our research.

No matter how advanced we are in our research endeavors, our learning stops when we think we know everything. Such closed mindedness is the complete opposite of the beginner's mind. When we were children, and we learned something new, everything felt fresh and new. For example, do you remember what it was like to learn to ride a bike? Everything was new; we saw the world from an exciting and fresh vantage point. We were thrilled with the feeling of the wind rushing through our hair. We were in awe of the new skill and what we learned. But now, years later, when we hop on our bikes, we have lost the ability to see and experience riding the bike for the first time simply because we have done it so many times. For most of us, after we grew up, we lost the ability to see and experience things with a beginner's mind. In doing so, we ended up losing the simple richness that used to underpin our day-to-day lives. Each moment should be characterized as fresh and new, but we bring so many thoughts and ideas into the moment that we often lose the ability to experience it with a beginner's mind.

DEVELOPING THE BEGINNER'S MIND

When was the last time you decided to learn something new? Maybe you had to learn a new software program for work, or your partner asked you to learn a new recipe to try in the kitchen, or you decided to try out a new exercise class with a friend. What was that experience like for you?

How did you feel before the experience? How did it make you feel after? What were you thinking and feeling throughout the experience? These reflection questions will provide insights into your thoughts, feelings, and experiences with developing a beginner's mind.

The beginner's mind is essential to increasing the richness of conducting interviews—a richer interview conversation results in more robust findings. This intentional mindset is also useful in overcoming the inevitable issues a researcher may face while collecting interview data.

THE INTERVIEW

To some extent, we interview every day of our lives. We ask our friends how the new restaurant was, what the weather may be, or we might ask our neighbors how they like the school their child attends. Asking questions to seek answers is natural to our communicative exchanges. However, using an interview for data collection is more intentional since the goal is to uncover specific pieces of information. Patton (2015) explains that:

We interview people to find out from them those things we cannot directly observe. . . . We cannot observe feelings, thoughts, and intentions. We cannot observe behaviors that took place at some previous point in time. We cannot observe situations that preclude the presence of an observer. We cannot observe how people have organized the world and the meanings they attach to what goes on in the world. We have to ask people questions about those things.

The purpose of interviewing, then, is to allow us to enter into the other person's perspective. (p. 426)

The ability to enter into another's perspective is a complex exchange. The exchange is intricate because both the inquirer and the inquired are fused together into a single reality in a single moment in time and knowledge derives from the exchange between the researcher and the participant (Lincoln, Lynham, & Guba, 2013). In this way, the two are linked and, therefore, interactive and inseparable (Lincoln & Guba, 1985). This inseparableness is magnified by the attitudes, biases, and preconceptions that both the participant and the researcher bring to the table. Because of the interconnectedness, the researcher has to work even harder to assess her stance and to exercise nonjudgment and sensitivity to the participant. This is a skill that comes with time, and researchers can often be unsure as to how to both identify and address preexisting knowledge, experience, and biases. I am reminded of one student in my graduate-level qualitative methods class who kept saying we have to remove biases. As a former journalist, it was hard for her to grasp that we don't remove biases, but rather acknowledge and adjust for them to ensure the quality of our data. This is one of the many skills that are necessary to overcome the challenges that may present themselves during the interview experience, which is underpinned by intricacies and nuance. For more specifics on how to approach the logistics of the long interview, see McCracken (1988).

Given the complexity of the interview process, let's take a closer look at some of the potential challenges a researcher may face while collecting data.

POTENTIAL INTERVIEW CHALLENGES

No matter how many times a researcher has conducted interviews, challenges will always present themselves. Since qualitative work deals with human beings, unpredictability and ambiguity are fundamental to the process. Specifically, researchers may have issues in dealing with distractions, not being able to record, remaining neutral, maintaining flexibility, and labeling the interview. Being aware of these issues is the first step. The second step is to apply the beginner's mind, which is developed through mindfulness, as an opportunity to address and circumvent these potential issues. Both are next.

Dealing With Distractions. Interviews demand the researcher pay attention and be present. However, distractions can detract from and impact a researcher's awareness. Technology has afforded researchers the ability to collect data in a different location than the participant, expanding reach and increasing the potential for sample variance. Yet the researcher needs to assess why interviews would be conducted over phone or video chat instead of in-person, since there are advantages and disadvantages of both (*see* Irvine, Drew, & Sainsbury, 2012). Beyond the advantages and disadvantages, distractions are inherent in both. In a phone interview, the participant cannot see what the researcher is doing, which means the researcher can be easily distracted. An email notification may ding, the phone ring, or a text come through, which immediately takes the researcher from the present moment to focus on the distraction. Although the distraction may only last for a split second, it takes the researcher away from the present moment shared with the participant. Even when interviews are held on a virtual platform, the researcher may face similar distractions that can take away from the conversation happening with the participant.

While the email window is easy to close and a phone can be put on silent, it is impossible to remove all distractions, which means a researcher needs to learn to let those distractions pass like clouds in the sky, and not to become attached to them. Being able to incorporate a beginner's mind in the interview process can assist with letting distractions pass because this perspective allows researchers to engage in the present moment with a heightened awareness that is rooted in being able to see things for the first time. So instead of hearing the email ding and then engaging in thoughts about who the email is from, what it could be about, and when you will be able to respond, you hear the ding, notice it, and then move right back to the present moment, letting the ding pass without getting caught up in all of the thought patterns we tend to associate with an email notification. This will help increase engagement in the present moment, which results in an enriching conversation with the participant.

While distractions exist with interviewing on technology, the in-person interview is not exempt from having similar interruptions. When in-person, the researcher may spend too much time taking notes and not engaging nonverbally with the participant, which could impact rapport building or the opportunity to probe on something the person said. In addition, the setting and subsequent background noise may end up being distracting.

I remember a time when I conducted an interview at the local coffee shop. Although it was a neutral and comfortable environment to meet and have a conversation with the participant, the background noise from the espresso machine and customers giving orders made it difficult to hear and pay attention. I had to really focus on my participant and try not to be distracted by the people walking in and out of the coffee shop and all of the commotion happening around us that was attempting to seize my senses. Even the audio recording was muffled because of the espresso machine and sidebar conversations. In some ways, this in-person interview was more difficult than one on the phone since paying attention in this setting was even more exhausting.

Similar to dealing with technological distractions, a beginner's mind can also assist in quickly navigating or avoiding in-person interview distractions. Let's take the previous example to illustrate. Had I been using my beginner's mind, I would have let those distractions pass like clouds, focusing on the uniqueness of the present moment with the participant. It would have allowed me to hit pause to hone into this brand-new experience (even though this was my 30th interview for this particular study). Seeing the participant and our conversation with fresh eyes and open ears would have allowed me to better block out the myriad of distractions that were present at the local coffee shop.

Not Being Able to Record. All researchers will face a time when the participant prefers not to be audio recorded but would like to be included in the study. This must be decided ahead of time and in compliance with the researcher's Institutional Review Board (IRB). When this happens, the researcher will be required to take notes, whether it be on a computer or by hand, while continuing the conversational nature of the interview. This situation requires a high level of active listening and attunement to the present moment; without it, nuance and insights will be missed, which is where the beginner's mind comes into play.

In this particular exchange, distractions have to be removed so that the participants' thoughts are captured while keeping the interview going in a conversational manner. Using the beginner's mind to let go of the thoughts associated with potential distractions helps keep the researcher in the present moment. In addition, contentment on capturing what is possible and not remaining attached to what is potentially missed is key. This contentment can be cultivated through the beginner's mind, where everything that is said is embraced and experienced as new and interesting, and the researcher doesn't get lost in what is missed or not captured. Most likely, if the information was important, it will show up again in another interview, and hopefully that interview can be captured using an audio recording device. Using the beginner's mind to cultivate a certain level of curiosity will help researchers overcome the frustrations that sometimes accompany this challenge. In welcoming this occasion with a beginner's mind, the participants can have a positive experience, where their thoughts are appropriately captured so they can be included in the study.

Remaining Neutral. In addition to dealing with different distractions and not being able to record, the level of neutrality exercised by the researcher also impacts the interview experience. Neutrality is essential in all data collection. Ideally, the researcher should remain neutral in response to the participants' beliefs and knowledge (Merriam & Tisdell, 2016). The interview often requires the participant to share personal information or experiences, and it is up to the interviewer to create a safe place for the participant to be willing to share personal information. In an interview, neutrality can be expressed through probes or nonverbal behavior such as head nodding (even when the interviewer may disagree), and not openly agreeing or disagreeing with the participant. Neutrality communicates to the participants that there are no right or wrong answers, but rather a chance simply to share their experiences, thoughts, and feelings without concern for getting it "right."

The beginner's mind helps us cultivate and apply neutrality when conducting interviews. Specifically, opening up our minds to the possibilities and beliefs that are beyond what we currently know and understand, we remove barriers to knowledge and insights. If the researcher is using preexisting knowledge to draw conclusions about the interview exchange, neutrality is lost, and the data could be tainted. Therefore, observing without judgment extends the possibilities of what information can be captured in an interview. Using the beginner's mind approach helps us make space in our minds for the things we don't know to avoid letting our preexisting information and assumptions guide the interview exchange.

Maintaining Flexibility. Maintaining flexibility needs to be exercised in the interview exchange; otherwise, challenges may present themselves. For example, a researcher may conduct an interview with someone who is not very talkative. This type of participant can be very difficult for the researcher because it is hard to elicit a response from a person who may be shy or introverted. Some people are not very loquacious or feel uncomfortable while being interviewed; the interview sometimes presents a level of formality that is hard to avoid. It is then up to the researcher to remain flexible in these situations, trying as many probing strategies as possible. What the researcher should not do is try to overcompensate by talking a lot more than the participant to fill in the gaps. Rather, the researcher should simply accept the interview for what it is and move on to the next one.

In other situations, the researcher may be faced with a distracted participant. For example, if an interview is being conducted in someone's home, there may be domestic distractions like partners, pets, or children. If the interview is conducted in someone's workplace, colleagues may come in and interrupt or the phone may ring, and the participant needs to answer it because the call is important. Therefore, a willingness to adapt and be flexible in these situations is essential.

Upholding such flexibility can be cultivated by having a beginner's mindset. When we characterize each interview as fresh and new, we are open to the experience as it unfolds, no matter what is happening in that moment. This level of openness leads to being flexible, to accepting any direction the conversation goes even if it is in an unanticipated direction. Seeing things anew with a beginner's mind also helps with the ever-changing nature of the qualitative research setting, which can oftentimes be driven by an emergent design, where things shift and change in real time. Welcoming such changes with a beginner's mind results in a heightened level of flexibility that allows the researcher to ebb and flow throughout the interview process no matter the situation.

Labeling the Interview. Any time we conduct human-participant research, issues are bound to arise given the unpredictability of human beings. This may lead the researcher to make initial assumptions about the quality of the interview and label it as either a *good* or *bad* interview. For example, one time I conducted an interview with a female executive who did not have much time for the interview. In general, high-profile people do not always have the ideal amount of time for an interview, but I was grateful for any amount of time she was willing to give. Throughout the interview, her answers seemed short and not as detailed compared to other participants in the study. Because of this, I initially labeled the interview in my mind as not very good due to the length of the conversation. However, after reviewing the transcript and recording, the interview was rich with details even though she spoke frankly and to the point. In the end, the interview did not uphold the initial label I assigned to it. From that moment on, I tried to exercise the practice of not labeling interviews and accepted the conversations as a contribution to data collection without assigning or labeling interviews with a particular quality.

The practice of nonlabeling is fundamental to the mindfulness practice and should be a tool incorporated by qualitative researchers through the beginner's mind. Labels are extensions of what is already known, and they help us make sense of the world. For adults, labels are used more frequently because of the number of previous experiences we rely on to make conclusions about those that may be similar in the present moment. However, children experience many things for the first time and lack the labels to make an assessment and draw a conclusion. Therefore, the beginner's mind helps a researcher see an interview like it is the first time, which helps avoid the desire and inclination to label the quality of the interview. The result is experiencing every interview with a fresh perspective—to be open to it as it unfolds, without making an assessment about its quality, but accepting exactly how it is in that moment.

The next section further explains a particular mindfulness practice that researchers should adapt to attune to the present moment to cultivate the beginner's mind while conducting interviews and navigating the potential issues that may arise.

THE PRACTICE: BODY SCAN

The best practice for honing the beginner's mind is the body scan, which is a Mindfulness-Based Stress Reduction (MBSR) meditation practice. Meditation is a great tool to reconnect with the beginner's mind, which is a renewed and refreshing state of awareness. Such awareness is key to overcoming interview challenges. The following body scan should first be done on a regular basis to get comfortable with the practice. Then the practice can be used routinely and before an actual interview. Setting aside 10 to 15 minutes will not only benefit you but will also create a positive experience for your participant. Shall we begin?

You will begin this body scan meditation by finding a quiet place to sit. You should find a place that you can sit in quietly, with an upright back, so you are active and alert, yet relaxed. Set your timer for 10 to 15 minutes and begin the meditation.

Start by sitting comfortably with a straight back. Close your eyes. You can place your hands in your lap or comfortably on your knees. Relax your neck and shoulders. Feel your body settle and relax into the seated posture. And as you begin to settle, start focusing on the breath. A calming or soothing breath, a breath that connects the mind and body. Notice how it draws into your body and how it leaves the body. Notice how you don't have to try to breathe, that it occurs naturally in the body. Use the breath to transition from where you just were to the present moment.

After you have spent a few moments in the breath, begin to expand your awareness to your body, paying attention to its entirety. Focus your attention on each part of the body. Start by bringing your attention to the top of your head and scalp. Feel whatever is happening in this area. You might feel strong sensations or nothing at all. The specifics are not important, but what is important is just recognizing what is there. Continue to move throughout the body from your scalp, to your face, to your shoulders, arms, and then the hands and fingers. Do you feel any itch, dryness, pulsing, or heat? You will then move your focus to your chest, back, and abdomen, continuing to the legs and finally to the feet and toes. If you feel any tension throughout, try to gently relax by using the breath to help it soften. We aren't trying to change any part of the experience or get anywhere— just see if you can observe things exactly as they are.

Throughout the entire body scan, each time you notice a sensation, recognize it. Experience it without thinking about it or labeling it. Get curious about it. If you notice any sensation, like warmth or coolness, tingling or pressure, tension or lightness, try to experience it as though it were the first time you have experienced this particular sensation. Observe it, but drop any commentary about the experience. See and sense the experience directly in and of itself. Notice each sensation as it rises and passes. As it rises, observe it without labeling it, without trying to change it. Simply notice what is there.

Once the timer goes off, notice how your mind and body feel. Do you feel relaxed? Have you created new space in your mind? Are you attuned to the present moment, ready to collect data? Complete your *Mindful Memos* by jotting down your thoughts, feelings, and sensations about the experience. The *Mindful Memos* will help capture how the mind shifts and changes over time.

CONCLUSION

This chapter provided an overview of the beginner's mind and how this mindset can be used by researchers. Interviews were discussed, as well as some challenges researchers may face while collecting data. The beginner's mind was woven throughout the interview challenges as a solution to potential hurdles. A mindfulness practiced was introduced—the body scan—as a means to develop the beginner's mindset. The body scan allows the practitioner to develop a new sense of curiosity about one's body without labeling the experience, which leads to the cultivation of the beginner's mind.

KEY TAKEAWAYS

- When we bring a beginner's mind to the research process, we stop being limited by our beliefs about others and instead see them as they really are: unique and interesting.

- The beginner's mind is essential to increasing the richness of conducting interviews—a richer interview conversation results in more robust findings.

- No matter how many times a researcher has conducted interviews, challenges will always present themselves. Specifically, researchers may have issues in dealing with distractions, not being able to record, remaining neutral, maintaining flexibility, and labeling the interview.

- To cultivate our beginner's mind, we need to engage in a practice. The best practice for honing this particular mindset is the body scan, which is a Mindfulness-Based Stress Reduction (MBSR) meditation practice.

- The body scan will be your practice for the next 2 weeks. Dedicate time each day to the body scan to see how you change and evolve over time, coming to the practice every day with an open mind.

REFLECTION QUESTIONS

- What excites you about conducting interviews? What concerns you about conducting interviews?

- Have you faced any challenges while conducting interviews? If so, what were those challenges?

- How can having a beginner's mind help you overcome challenges and concerns?

TWO-WEEK PRACTICE: THE BODY SCAN

The body scan will be your practice for the next 2 weeks. Dedicate time each day to the body scan to see how you change and evolve over time, coming to the practice every day with an open mind. Be sure to do your *Mindful Memos* at the end of each session. The memos are an incredible opportunity to capture how your mind will actually transform over the course of the practice. The meditation will get easier each time you sit, and soon enough you will rediscover your beginner's mind.

Mindful Memos

REFERENCES

Irvine, A., Drew, P., & Sainsbury, R. (2013). "Am I not answering your questions properly?" Clarification, adequacy and responsiveness in semi-structured telephone and face-to-face interviews. *Qualitative Research, 13*(1), 87–106.

Lincoln Y. S., & Guba, E. G. (1985). *Naturalistic inquiry.* Sage.

Lincoln, Y. S., Lynham, S. A., & Guba, E. G. (2013). Paradigmatic controversies, contradictions, and emerging confluences, revisited. In *The landscape of qualitative research* (4th ed.). Sage.

McCracken, Grant. (1988). *The long interview.* Sage.

Merriam, S. B., & Tisdell, E. J. (2016). *Qualitative research: A guide to design and implementation* (4th ed.). Jossey-Bass.

Patton, M. Q. (2015). *Qualitative research and evaluation methods* (4th ed.). Sage.

SHARING LOVING-KINDNESS IN FOCUS GROUPS

4

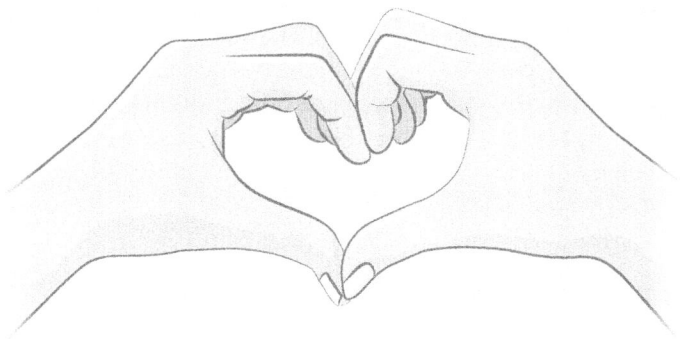

This chapter, Sharing Loving-Kindness in Focus Groups, introduces the loving-kindness meditation as a tool to prepare for moderating focus groups. The loving-kindness approach is about exercising self-compassion, offering understanding toward yourself, and extending it to those around you. This statement might prompt you to think: What exactly does this have to do with focus groups? Focus groups are unique in that confidentiality is impossible, and in some cases, the participants are not entirely familiar with the other people in the group. Therefore, to help facilitate a successful conversation among focus group participants, a certain level of respect needs to be shared to ensure everyone feels comfortable speaking up and communicating their insights and experiences. This level of care and respect starts with the moderator or researcher. To demonstrate respect and care for others, we must first learn how to show that level of compassion with ourselves.

Empathy and understanding are necessary when we engage in qualitative research, where the focus is on the participants and researcher coming together, sharing space, and engaging in a conversation—this is especially true for focus groups. When we show compassion and understanding to ourselves, we are able to exhibit those same considerations to others. If we do not show ourselves the same level of empathy, we do not have the ability to show others kindness and compassion. Such levels of compassion, understanding, and kindness are required in the research setting, especially with focus groups. These qualities are going to propel us to the next level in our research and in our lives.

This chapter begins with an overview of the loving-kindness meditation, which is followed by a summary of focus groups and their benefits. This chapter transitions into the challenges a researcher may have to navigate and how the loving-kindness meditation can assist in this journey. The next section describes how to carry out the loving-kindness meditation. Pages for the *Mindful Memos* conclude the chapter.

WHAT IS THE LOVING-KINDNESS MEDITATION?

The loving-kindness meditation is a unique approach to meditation that focuses on cultivating unconditional attitudes of kindness to oneself and others by concentrating attention on certain groups of people and silently repeating four caring phrases such as *may you be healthy; may you be happy; may you be safe*; and *may you be at peace* (Zeng et al., 2015). The people the meditator focuses on change over the course of the meditation, moving from the self, to a loved one, to a difficult person, and to an entire community, with special emphasis on showing compassion to each person or group of people.

Recent research studies have demonstrated the positive impact of consistently engaging in a mindfulness practice that includes the loving-kindness meditation. For example, Galante et al. (2014) conducted a meta-analysis of existing research and found that the loving-kindness meditation can cultivate positive emotions. Shonin et al. (2015) also concluded that the loving-kindness meditation can significantly improve positive emotional states. Specifically, a consistent loving-kindness meditation can decrease depression and rumination, in addition to improving positive emotions (Shonin et al., 2015).

Before covering how the loving-kindness meditation can be a useful tool for focus groups, let's briefly discuss the role of these groups in qualitative data collection.

THE FOCUS GROUP

Focus groups are a qualitative method that relies on group interaction. The explicit group collaboration produces data and subsequent insights that are only possible through the engagement among group members (Morgan, 1997). Specifically, focus groups bring "together a group, or, more often, a series of groups, of subjects to discuss an issue in the presence of a moderator" (Lunt & Livingstone, 1996, p. 80). In this way, the focus group becomes a socially positioned conversation among the participants, where the goal is to generate a discussion that may occur in everyday life (1996). These groups can be small or large, and the conversations can be directed or nondirected depending on the research questions and needs of the study (Kamberelis & Dimitriadis, 2013).

Benefits of Focus Groups. Data collection using focus groups provides a myriad of opportunities for the researcher. First, the focus group provides the researcher the ability to collect large amounts of data quickly—more so than an interview, and more specific than participant observation (Morgan, 1997).

Second, focus groups provide space for both the individual and the collective to engage in conversation about a given topic (Kamberelis & Dimitriadis, 2013). An individual can share experiences with the collective to see if others have similar or even dissimilar experiences. This space is especially helpful in giving a voice to marginalized groups of people, encouraging them to share their experiences and insights (2013). For example, participatory action research projects may rely heavily on such approaches to promote conversation and potential liberation among the group members, since the priority is for all group members to come alongside the researcher to cultivate actionable change. Focus groups can be a place for "transformation, collective action, and the possibility of examining the self and other in different ways" (Swaminathan, 2017, p. 54).

Third, focus groups encourage a dialogic openness that may not have been possible in an interview or participant observation (Lunt & Livingstone, 1996). Although the moderator is present in the focus groups, the positioning of the researcher is less prominent in the conversation than in, for example, an interview, which may lead to a deeper conversation among the participants—here, there is power in numbers, where the conversation among the focus group participants can uncover insightful details. The emphasis is on the group as a collective versus a set of individuals (Swaminathan, 2017). In addition, when people share experiences that others can relate to, the dialogue among participants leads to a collective vulnerability shared, respected, and honored by all. The results are rich data that stem from the engaging social interactions.

Despite the benefits that focus groups provide, the researcher needs to be prepared to handle potential challenges. With all research, preparing for and being open to the unknown will help us adapt and respond in real time to the situations or issues that may be present during data collection. The next section addresses some of the potential challenges that may arise when conducting focus groups, using some of my previous experiences to illustrate.

USING THE LOVING-KINDNESS MEDITATION TO NAVIGATE POTENTIAL FOCUS GROUP CHALLENGES

Challenges are inherent in all research, and focus groups are no exception. Depending on the participants in the focus group or the questions asked, more challenges arise. This section will address some of these potential obstacles a researcher will face when collecting data via focus groups. Specifically, this section covers challenges related to sensitive topics, active listening, groupthink, and lack of anonymity. I would like to point out that barriers are not always inherently negative, but rather just a characteristic of the qualitative research process. Additionally, this section provides details as to how incorporating a loving-kindness meditation can help the researcher navigate some of the obstacles unique to focus groups.

Discussing Sensitive Topics. The first challenge deals with conducting research that covers sensitive topics. Focus groups provide an opportunity for like-minded people to engage in a conversation. Oftentimes, these conversations address difficult issues and encounters. These discussions can lead to a certain level of liberation and understanding for participants because there is power in people coming together to discuss similar shared, lived experiences.

Participatory action research and critical scholarship often rely on focus groups to bring people together to share meaningful, yet sometimes difficult experiences (Kamberelis & Dimitriadis, 2013). For example, a critical scholar may rely on focus groups to gather women's experiences in dealing with misogyny and discrimination that stem from a patriarchal workplace. During the focus group, the moderator would most likely ask the participants to share about particular experiences they have been involved with in the workplace. This may prompt participants to exercise a high level of vulnerability in sharing personal information. Without a skilled moderator who makes participants feel welcomed, ensures trust, and creates an inclusive environment, encouraging participants to share their personal experiences may be difficult.

This is where a loving-kindness meditation can help the moderator prepare for the focus group. Although the value of the focus group is the insight that comes from the shared experience, creating a space that cultivates these tough conversations requires empathy and understanding on behalf of the moderator. The loving-kindness meditation can help the moderator prepare for difficult yet meaningful conversations since the nature of the meditation is to extend care and understanding to the self and others. This practice helps set the tone for the focus group, which often begins with the moderator. It can also help the moderator attune to the present moment, which is discussed next.

Exercising Active Listening. The second issue deals with the active presence of the moderator. The role of the researcher is unique in the focus group in that the moderator is the conversation starter but not the main speaker in the conversation. This is different than the interview, where the participant and researcher engage together, with the researcher guiding the conversation. In focus groups, the participants engage with each other, and the moderator is separate from the conversation. Although the moderator asks the questions, the goal is to facilitate the conversation *among*, not with, the participants. This requires an acute attention to the present moment, following the conversation as it emerges.

To be able to facilitate a conversation among a group of people requires a special kind of attention—active listening. Ethical, active listening has several key elements such as demonstrating recognition, acknowledging others, paying attention, communicating fairly, giving consideration to all viewpoints, and responding appropriately and with respect (Macnamara, 2016).

Active listening results from being able to exercise acute attention to the unfolding conversation among the focus group participants. It is a balancing act between reviewing the guide, using nonverbal cues, following the conversation, and interjecting when necessary to keep the discussion relevant to the study's topic. Interjections need to be done with finesse, where the moderator does not impact the group dynamic by asking others to share or moving on from a topic that wasn't fully discussed. All these skills require an attunement to the present moment.

Being an active listener is a special skill that is developed and perfected over time. It starts with being present, showing each person in the focus group that you are engaged and interested in what they have to say. If the moderator sets the tone of actively paying attention with what is happening at that moment, the rest of the focus group will hopefully follow suit. One way to practice this skill is to incorporate the loving-kindness meditation in a daily routine. This meditation helps the researcher learn how to focus on and be active in the present moment. This leads to developing the necessary skills required of being an active listener.

One Person Dominating the Conversation. The moderator's or the participants' attention can become distracted or compromised when one participant begins to dominate the conversation, which is the third potential issue that a focus group moderator may face. In general, the conversation should flow freely in a focus group. However, times will arise when the moderator needs to call on a specific person to ensure the participant is part of the conversation. There will also be situations when one particular person dominates the conversation. This can be problematic because it discourages others from sharing their thoughts, opinions, or experiences. Therefore, the moderator will have to find a strategic way to invite others into the conversation without offending the person who is dominating the conversation.

To elaborate, I was moderating a focus group for a multibillion-dollar defense contractor for the government and faced with a situation where one gentleman dominated the conversation. He had just experienced an unfortunate situation, where the organization changed his pension and benefits after nearly 30 years with the company. Needless to say, he was not pleased. The focus group gave him a chance to air his grievances and be heard in a place where there were no repercussions for his honesty. As a matter of fact, this is one of the principal benefits of focus groups and for all qualitative research. Often, focus groups provide people a voice who may have felt unheard or silenced; there is liberation in feeling you have finally been heard. In fact, one woman began to cry as she expressed similar experiences and feelings of being undervalued. By demonstrating care, participants will feel comfortable enough to share their frustrations and confidences. The balance is about making sure people feel heard, while welcoming insights and opinions from others.

Exercising care to someone who may be dominating the conversation is a great way for the moderator to navigate this situation. Using the same principles developed in the loving-kindness meditation, such as care and understanding, the moderator can skillfully and kindly work with a person who may be dominating the discussion. It ensures this person feels heard, yet welcomes and encourages others to join in.

Navigating Groupthink. When conducting focus groups, the moderator needs to be aware of the potential for groupthink and work to prevent group bias among the participants, which is the fourth potential challenge. In my research experiences, I have faced groupthink, which was a bit tricky to navigate. Groupthink is when participants conform and even censor their responses based on what others in the group are saying (MacDougall & Baum, 1997). When groupthink occurs, not all perspectives are shared and the conversation among participants is not as rich. This does not mean that the group cannot agree on a particular perspective—instead, the goal is to gather and welcome as many differing perspectives as possible.

In the study I discussed above, I was interested in capturing participants' experiences with employee engagement and internal communication in the midst of major organizational changes, which is something that happens frequently with government contractors. In one focus group, people started talking about the changes and issues related to their healthcare benefits. Since I am not a human resources scholar, this was not the focus of my study. However, through the conversation, participants began discussing their concerns and disappointments with the benefit changes. This conversation deviated from the focus group guide, yet the participants were incredibly passionate about sharing their experiences. I was between a rock and a hard place (an appropriate cliché metaphor). I had to tactfully recognize their thoughts, feelings, and concerns, while slowly drifting the conversation back to the topic(s) of the study. This took some time, which was appropriate, so the participants did not feel as though it was an abrupt change. Slowly, but surely, I was able to shift the conversation back to questions from the guide without hurting people's feelings or making them feel as though they were being cut off from sharing.

Although groupthink may be helpful in some research projects, times may occur when it is not helpful in advancing the phenomenon under investigation. The moderator will have to slowly and sensitively guide the conversation back to a discussion related to the research topic. If done too abruptly, participants may feel as though the moderator is exhibiting power over the group. Embarking on such an endeavor using a loving-kindness mentality will make sure the participants are not put off or offended by having to transition away from a topic about which they feel passionately.

Addressing Anonymity. Although focus groups function in a way that decenters the researcher to give participants control and ownership (Kamberelis & Dimitriadis, 2013), the researcher still needs to set the tone for how people approach and treat others in the group. This is especially true since anonymity is not possible, and confidentiality needs to be upheld, which is the last focus group challenge. To ensure this level of trust is established among focus group participants, the moderator needs to set the group rules before the conversation starts. These ground rules should be rooted in respect and demonstrate loving-kindness for members of the group. Below is a list of some of the ground rules I use to begin focus groups.

FOCUS GROUP GROUND RULES

- There are no right or wrong answers. I only want to know your thoughts and opinions, and every opinion is valuable.
- I would ask that you respect everyone's confidentiality by not sharing what you hear today outside of this room.
- It is important that only one person speaks at a time, and we all listen and show respect while that person is speaking.
- You do not have to speak in any particular order. The goal is to have a free-flowing conversation.
- When you do have something to say, please do so. There are many of you in the group, and it is important that I obtain the views of each of you.
- You do not have to agree with the views of other people in the group.

Using the ground rules can be helpful, especially when it comes to addressing anonymity and confidentiality. This allows the participants to know how they will be treated and how to treat others, which is vital when people are sharing personal information. For example, I was conducting focus groups with students to better understand their experiences with crowdfunding and willingness to become donors after graduating from the university. The focus group participants knew each other to varying degrees since they were all students at the same university within the same college. After covering the ground rules, I began asking the participants to share their experiences. Yet the conversation was stifled at the beginning. This was partially due to the power dynamics, with the students feeling uncomfortable sharing. I knew that I needed to reiterate the ground rules by focusing on the confidentiality piece and emphasizing the value of everyone's contribution. This helped ease some of the tension so that the conversation could begin. Slowly, but surely, the participants shared what was on their minds in response to the questions asked.

Given the discussion of some challenges a focus group moderator may face, the next section further explains the loving-kindness approach to increase presence with and compassion for participants, creating a welcoming space for all participants to engage in respectful dialogue.

THE PRACTICE: LOVING-KINDNESS MEDITATION

Focus groups often address difficult questions that require a certain level of vulnerability within the group. As mentioned earlier, the group's willingness to be vulnerable is cultivated by the moderator. The moderator should have a strong sense of loving-kindness and compassion to the self so that the same sympathies can be given to those in the focus group, resulting in the participants sharing this same affinity with each other. It begins with showing compassion toward the self, which is cultivated through a loving-kindness mindfulness practice.

We often discuss sharing loving-kindness to others, but interestingly enough, we find it difficult to offer it to ourselves. We are hard on ourselves and demand perfection. This is particularly true for academic scholars. The demands of the job often cause imposter syndrome and a constant striving for perfection. Therefore, we do not always show the same compassion for ourselves that we show toward others. It takes practice to show this kind of compassion, and meditation is a way to identify our tendencies to talk poorly to ourselves. If any of us paid attention to the voices we all had in our heads, we would probably hear constant judgment. We would never allow our friends, family, or colleagues to speak to us this way. But for some reason, we put up with it in ourselves. When we do not show ourselves compassion, offering it to others is difficult.

The following loving-kindness meditation should be done on a regular basis to gain experience, and then before moderating a focus group. Setting aside 10 to 15 minutes will not only benefit you but also create a positive experience for the participants in the room. Let us begin to see how exuding compassion toward ourselves and others feels.

You will begin this loving-kindness meditation by finding a quiet place to sit. You should find a place where you can sit quietly, with an upright back, so you are active and alert, yet relaxed. Set your timer for 10 to 15 minutes and begin the meditation.

Start by sitting comfortably, with a straight back. Close your eyes. You can place your hands in your lap or comfortably on your knees. Relax your neck and shoulders. Unwind your jaw. Feel your body settle and relax. And as you begin to settle, start focusing on the breath. A calming or soothing breath, a breath that connects the mind and body. Notice how it draws into your body and how it leaves the body. Allow the breath to transition from where you just were to the present moment. Mentally note when you are breathing in and when you are breathing out. Each time you breathe in, welcome the next breath. When you release it, do so with openness. As you breathe, do so without judgment. Accept all that may come up as you breathe into the present moment. Spend a few minutes simply focusing on the breath.

Now that you have settled, using the breath to anchor into the present moment, let's transition to generating loving-kindness toward ourselves. Begin to offer yourself a feeling of friendliness and gentleness. Breathe in and out while showing compassion to the self.

Let's transition to practice some standard phrases of loving-kindness. They could include: *May I be happy. May I be healthy. May I be safe. May I be at peace.* These are not affirmations, where we are trying to convince ourselves of anything; instead, we should welcome and accept them as gifts. You can use these phrases or any that come to mind and resonate most with you personally. Use the same phrases every time or switch up the phrases that you select to use. I encourage you to try out different phrases to see which ones resonate the most with you. Remember, there are no "right" or "wrong" phrases; they are simply statements that offer a compassionate kindness we all deserve. Pick four statements that are most meaningful to you. Continue to repeat your chosen four phrases at a pace that feels comfortable.

The next phrase is to now offer the same loving-kindness to someone you care about. This person makes you happy the moment you think of them. Picture that person and hold them in your awareness. Once you get a feeling for their loving presence, extend loving-kindness toward them. It can be more than one person, if you'd like, extending kindness to anyone who warms your heart. Repeat the same phrases while thinking of that person(s): *May they be happy. May they be healthy. May they be safe. May they be at peace.*

Now, we extend loving-kindness toward a neutral person. Perhaps it is a colleague, a stranger, or even your focus group participant(s). Visualize that person or persons in your mind and show them loving-kindness by repeating the following phrases: *May they be happy. May they be healthy. May they be safe. May they be at peace.*

The last is to extend loving-kindness to all beings. You can focus your attention on the people in your community or all over the world. Extend affection without boundaries or limits, spreading loving-kindness in all directions. Repeat the same phrases to show warm wishes to everyone: *May all beings be happy. May all beings be healthy. May all beings be safe. May all beings be at peace.*

Once the timer goes off, notice how it feels to open the heart and generate loving-kindness with the self and others. Can you see a shift in the compassion you showed yourself? Will this feeling of compassion transcend into data collection? How can you bring loving-kindness into the research setting? Spend a few minutes recording your thoughts, feelings, and sensations about the experience in your *Mindful Memos*.

The loving-kindness meditation will be your practice for the next 2 weeks. Dedicate time each day to this meditation to see how you change and evolve over time, coming to the practice every day with an open mind. Be sure to complete the *Mindful Memos* at the end of each session, so you can capture the changes you may experience over the 2 weeks. The loving-kindness meditation allows you to experience more compassion and understanding for yourself and those around you.

CONCLUSION

The purpose of this chapter was to introduce how the loving-kindness meditation can be used to help the moderator prepare for focus groups and navigate challenges that may arise. The chapter covered some of the obstacles the researcher will have to address when using focus groups to collect data. Also included in the chapter are an overview of the loving-kindness meditation and detailed instructions on how to engage in the practice.

KEY TAKEAWAYS

- The chapter introduced the loving-kindness meditation as a tool to prepare for moderating focus groups.

- The loving-kindness approach is about exercising self-compassion, offering understanding toward yourself, and then extending it to those around you by silently repeating four caring phrases.

- Using the loving-kindness meditation can help the researcher navigate challenges that may arise in moderating focus groups such as discussing sensitive topics, actively listening, circumventing groupthink, and addressing anonymity.

- The loving-kindness meditation practice helps us learn how to cultivate self-compassion, which can then be transferred to our focus group participants.

REFLECTION QUESTIONS

- How does it feel to show yourself compassion? What about it is easy? What about it is difficult?

- How can the feelings of kindness and compassion transcend into moderating focus groups? What roadblocks or challenges might make this difficult?

- What other ways can you bring loving-kindness into the research setting?

TWO-WEEK PRACTICE: LOVING-KINDNESS MEDITATION

The loving-kindness meditation will be your practice for the next 2 weeks. Dedicate time each day to the loving-kindness meditation to see how you change and evolve over time, coming to the practice every day with an open mind. Be sure to do your *Mindful Memos* at the end of each session. The memos are an incredible opportunity to capture how your mind will actually transform over the course of the practice. The meditation will get easier each time you sit, and soon enough you will refine your ability to show and accept loving-kindness.

Mindful Memos

_____

_____

_____

_____

_____

_____

_____

_____

_____

_____

_____

_____

_____

_____

_____

_____

_____

_____

_____

_____

_____

_____

_____

_____

REFERENCES

Galante, J., Galante, I., Bekkers, M. J., & Gallacher, J. (2014). Effect of kindness-based meditation on health and well-being: A systematic review and meta-analysis. *J. Consult. Clin. Psychol. 82*, 1101–1114. https://doi.org/10.1037/a0037249

Kamberelis, G., & Dimitriadis, G. (2013). Focus groups. In N. K. Denzin & Y. S. Lincoln (Eds.), *Collecting and interpreting qualitative materials* (4th ed., pp. 309–344). Sage.

Lunt, P., & Livingstone, S. (1996). Rethinking the focus group in media and communication research. *Journal of Communication, 46*, 79–97.

MacDougall, C., & Baum, F. (1997). The devil's advocate: A strategy to avoid groupthink and stimulate discussion in focus groups. *Qualitative Health Research* 7(4), 532–541. https://doi.org/10.1177/104973239700700407

Macnamara, J. (2016). Organizational listening: Addressing a major gap in public relations theory and practice. *Journal of Public Relations Research, 28*, 1–24. https://doi.org/10.1080/1062726X.2016.1228064

Morgan, D. L. (1997). *Focus groups as qualitative research* (2nd ed.). Sage.

Shonin, E., Van Gordon, W., Compare, A., Zangeneh, M., & Griffiths, M. D. (2015). Buddhist-derived loving-kindness and compassion meditation for the treatment of psychopathology: A systematic review. *Mindfulness, 6*, 1161–1180. https://doi.org/10.1007/s12671-014-0368-1

Swaminathan, R., & Mulvihill, T. M. (2017). *Critical approaches to questions in qualitative research*. Taylor & Francis.

Zeng, X., Chiu, C. P., Wang, R., Oei, T. P., & Leung, F. Y. (2015). The effect of loving-kindness meditation on positive emotions: A meta-analytic review. *Frontiers in Psychology, 6*, 1–14. https://doi.org/10.3389/fpsyg.2015.01693

MINDFULLY WALKING INTO PARTICIPANT OBSERVATION

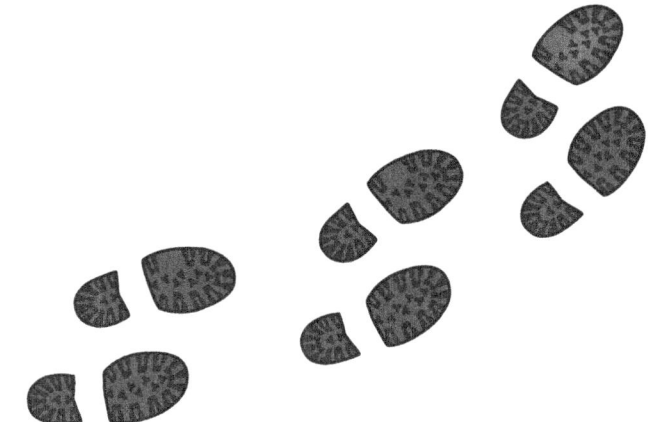

This chapter, Mindfully Walking Into Participant Observation, begins by introducing the walking meditation and how it relies on all five senses. The chapter then overviews participant observation and subsequent challenges a researcher may face while in the field. The chapter explains how using all five senses will help the researcher prepare to enter the field, improve observation skills, and address data collection challenges. The chapter transitions into how to complete the walking meditation, a practice that promotes the use of all five senses. It ends with a conclusion, key takeaways, and reflection questions. A space for the *Mindful Memos* is included along with a summary of the practice.

WALKING MEDITATION TO OBSERVE OUR FIVE SENSES

The previous chapters in this book have focused on attuning to the present moment in the traditional sense since the practices have focused on different approaches to a sitting meditation. This chapter shifts to a more action-based meditation that includes actual walking. In doing so, we are taking our meditation to the streets so we can easily incorporate it into our daily life. Additionally, the practice is going to amplify our consciousness to use our other senses, not just listening. We have spent weeks with our eyes closed. Now, we are going to open our eyes to the world around us and use the walking meditation to enhance our awareness of the five senses.

Research has demonstrated the value and impact of engaging in a walking meditation over time. For example, Gianey et al. (2016) found that patients with type 2 diabetes experienced a reduction in cortisol and blood glucose levels after participating in a 12-week walking meditation class. In fact, the participants experienced more benefits from the walking meditation program compared to a traditional walking plan (2016). An additional study discovered that a walking meditation practice improved adolescents' ability to express emotions (Kim & Ki, 2014). Similarly, Edwards, Rosenbaum, and Loprinzi (2017) found that walking meditation positively impacts the lives of young adults by observing that a consistent practice can improve anxiety states.

The walking meditation is unique in that it helps us develop all five senses: sound, touch, sight, taste, and smell. This practice is about awakening all of the senses to prepare for the research setting. Specifically, the walking meditation is going to be useful in collecting observational data, which requires all five senses to work in concert so that the research setting comes alive.

Principally, we use our senses without totally being aware we are employing them. For example, when was the last time you ate a meal while scrolling social media or watching television? My guess is that you finished your meal and did not even remember eating it, let alone actually tasted the food. Or maybe you walked to the store or mailbox but were thinking about your day and missed the sights, sounds, and smells that accompanied you on your walk. By tuning into our five senses, we experience present moments in vivid detail. It is almost as if you are moving from seeing things in black and white to viewing the world in technicolor.

Imagine what is missed in collecting field data if the senses are not recognized and utilized. What nuance is missed because we are only operating with sound or sight? Detailed descriptions of what is being observed is the value of observational data. But observations should encompass more than what is seen. It includes capturing what sounds are heard, what smells fill the air, what tactile sensations are felt, and even what certain tastes are experienced, especially if food and drink accompany the research context. In practicing the walking meditation prior to data collection, the researcher brings awareness to the five senses so that all of these unique elements are captured. Heightened awareness can also help the researcher navigate participant observation challenges.

Before we discuss how the walking meditation can enliven the senses in the field to navigate potential issues, let's talk briefly about how we can work on noticing our five senses. The exercise is called 5-4-3-2-1. It only takes a minute or two, but it will help us begin to notice and pay attention to our senses. The first step is to *see* five items in your surrounding area. Just look around you in this moment—what five items do you see? Now, let's *touch* four items. Again, pick four items in your immediate vicinity to touch. Next, pick out three *sounds.* The sounds can be close by or far away. Up next is *smell*—what two smells are you experiencing in this moment? Last is *taste*, and only focuses on one taste. What do you taste at this very moment? The 5-4-3-2-1 exercise is a great tool to begin a walking meditation. It is also a great resource to ground you in the present moment while collecting participant observation data, especially if you feel as though you are getting overwhelmed or distracted.

THE 5-4-3-2-1 EXERCISE WITH EXAMPLES

Pick out five things you can see (trees, animals, loved ones, books, computer).

Identify four things you can touch (keyboard, pen, water bottle, cell phone, plants).

Find three things you can hear (lawn mower, dishwasher, cars, television, music).

Pinpoint two things you can smell (food, coffee, cleaning solution, laundry, flowers).

Detect one taste (breakfast, toothpaste, ChapStick, water, tea).

PARTICIPANT OBSERVATION

Participant observation is a great tool to collect primary data, especially in case study and ethnographic research, where firsthand observation is desired. Additionally, this method for data collection is useful when participants may not feel entirely comfortable discussing a particular topic. This is especially true for observations that include online communication, since this medium provides an opportunity for participants to be included who may be reluctant to contribute directly (Angrosino & Rosenberg, 2013). Participant observation collects data in real time and can provide an in-depth context that leads to insights about interpersonal motives and behavior (Yin, 2018). The descriptive nature of the method is also helpful for bringing the voices of marginalized communities to the forefront, where the observations can help illuminate social justice issues and raise the consciousness of various research communities (Angrosino & Rosenberg, 2013).

However, this technique is different than the previously discussed interviews and focus groups for two primary reasons. First, the researcher conducts an observation in the location in which the phenomenon is naturally occurring (Merriam & Tisdell, 2016). Second, the data collected represent a firsthand observation of the phenomenon instead of a secondhand interpretation of what previously occurred (Merriam & Tisdell, 2016). Here, the distance between the observer and the observed lessens, and the two become co-creators in the research process (Angrosino & Rosenberg, 2013).

Participant observation requires the researcher to rely on the five senses to capture what is going on in the present moment. Field notes are used to capture not only what the researcher sees but also what is heard, felt, smelt, and even, in some cases, tasted. For example, DeSantis (2002) observed a local cigar shop in order to better understand why anti-smoking messages were unsuccessful in convincing customers to stop smoking. To collect data, DeSantis was first considered a regular and, therefore, became a trusted observer, gaining access to the rituals and conversations among shop customers. Data collection included interviews but also detailed descriptions of significant events, which captured what he saw, smelt, tasted, felt, and heard given that smoking cigars at the local cigar shop was a multisensory experience. The multisensory experience led to rich data that helped to uncover why this particular sample population was dismissive of anti-smoking messaging and engaged in pro-smoking communication exchanges. To be clear, I am not advocating for participating in behaviors that are harmful to your health but use this as an example to illustrate how collecting data from participant observation often includes all of the five senses. The results are data steeped in thick description that bring a certain context or phenomenon to life, which is the value of participant observation.

Participant observation does attract some disapproval since it is considered to be highly subjective, and therefore potentially unreliable (Merriam & Tisdell, 2016). However, some argue that although there is an element of subjectivity, strategic and rigorous observation is not so subjective that it cannot count as viable data (Angrosino & Rosenberg, 2013). To overcome the subjectivity criticism, mental preparation and training are key so that the researcher can become a capable and thorough observer. Training may include learning how to pay attention to what matters, systematically observe details, develop a system to record descriptive field notes, and incorporate methods to triangulate the observed insights (Patton, 2015).

POTENTIAL PARTICIPANT OBSERVATION CHALLENGES

Despite the many values that accompany field work and participant observation, challenges do present themselves. A few challenges include knowing when and how to enter the field, becoming overloaded with observation data, and recognizing when insider blindness is taking over. These encounters are discussed next in conjunction with suggestions on how the walking meditation with heightened senses can help navigate such issues.

Entering the Field. Participant observation is somewhat ambiguous in nature (Merriam & Tisdell, 2016), where the researcher is a bit unsure as to when to begin collecting data, what should be recognized as data, and how involved the researcher should be in the data collection process. Merriam and Tisdell (2016) refer to these ambiguities as "schizophrenic" activities since there is this push and pull of being involved in what is observed but not to the extent that total absorption occurs (p. 146).

When I conducted a case study of a particularly large client, it was difficult in the beginning to know when I was "entering the field" in terms of starting to collect data, which data I should be focusing on, and how involved I was to be in the process. For example, to begin my days, I had to visit a security checkpoint to acquire my visitor badge for the day. I was technically onsite, but was this part of my data collection? Should I be capturing my interactions with the security staff? Were these important data that would inform my study on internal communication and employee engagement? Ultimately, I made the executive decision that the answer to these questions was no. I was not engaging with communication professionals, the security folks were following a daily routine to admit visitors, and I was not observing data relevant to my study. However, when the communication professionals who were my points of contact met me at the security station, and I was able to observe their interactions with the security people, *those* were data. I wrote down those observations in my field notes because they provided insight into how the communication professionals within this organization interacted with other employees.

Another element of complexity with participant observation is the ability to collect data online. With technological advancements in the

21st century, we have the option to enter a virtual community. A virtual community is constructed through computer-meditated communication and online interactions among members (Angrosino & Rosenberg, 2013). Despite their value and commonplace occurrence, online communication and observations do have challenges. First, the observations are based solely on the written expressions and/or consciously selected images or videos by participants (Angrosino & Rosenberg, 2013). Second, the conversations lack the nonverbal communication like body language and gestures that help the researcher make sense of the communicative exchange (Angrosino & Rosenberg, 2013). This requires the researcher to uncover the potentially nuanced connotations and online communication strategies prior to the observations. The researcher needs to decide upfront how involved they want to be in the online community. Do they disclose who they are? Do they engage in promoted interactions with online community members, or do they quietly observe? Again, these questions can be difficult to answer, but they must be addressed before entering the field.

Participating in a walking meditation to observe and engage with the world around us is helpful in making decisions about entering the field. This particular meditation practice turns on our senses so that we are cognizant of our surroundings—more so than we usually are, which makes this a unique technique to help researchers prepare for the field. By participating in a walking meditation, we can get clarity on the questions that need to be addressed before entering the field in addition to being prepared to respond to questions that arise when collecting data.

Observation Overload. The second challenge a researcher may face with participant observation is how much data should be captured and the process for recording data. Upon entering the field, a researcher may have a sense of not wanting to miss anything because it *could* be important or feel as though there is too much going on to know what count as data. However, researchers have to establish boundaries to their observations. This delicate dance of collecting enough data so the details are captured, but not too much where it is hard to uncover what is most valuable, can be a challenge for researchers. Completing a walking meditation prior to entering the field can help the researcher prepare for these trials.

Interestingly, by awakening the five senses, we are able to slow our heart rate down and begin to focus on the present moment. We learn to focus on the details, but not complicate them. This active meditation also helps us learn how to respond to the world around us and trust that what we observe is enough. If something is missed in data collection, we also know that the emergent nature of field work means the insight will present itself again in subsequent observations.

The other challenge associated with observation overload is figuring out what to actually write down. Recording data onsite and in online environments can range from continuous recording data to scribbled notes to not recording anything until the researcher has left the field (Merriam & Tisdell, 2016). The recording process needs to be decided upon upfront by the researcher, and the walking meditation can be key in helping the researcher figure out the best approach. Following an interactive walking meditation, the researcher can decide what will be the best approach to collect data once in the field. Additionally, the researcher will want to tap into all five senses during observations to avoid being only dependent on sight. The research setting will come alive in the thick descriptions that capture what was felt, heard, smelt, and tasted, in addition to what was seen.

Insider Limitations. Being an insider within a culture under investigation can provide certain advantages such as a deeper level of understanding, established relationships with the social actors, quicker rapport-building, and potentially more open and honest conversations. For example, one of the reasons why the previously discussed study on cigar smokers was successful was the author was a regular to the cigar shop prior to data collection, giving him insider access (DeSantis, 2002). Similarly, Taylor's (2011) research on queer culture and sexual identity was an accessible research setting since the author was personally involved with the community for more than a decade, developing friendships with many members. This allowed for honest conversations about very personal topics and access to events that the average person/researcher would not be invited to attend (Taylor, 2011).

Despite the many values of being an insider in conducting participant observations, there are some downfalls, which researchers seldom discuss (Taylor, 2011). The first is that the researcher may not recognize the norms and rituals that have become second nature (Tracy, 2020). Data distortion can also occur, where only the good are observed and recorded, and the bad are minimized or not acknowledged. The insider perspective can also lead to role displacement, where the researcher crosses the line between researcher and active participant, which can impact professional conduct. Last, the connections and relationships made prior to or during the research process may be impacted (Taylor, 2011).

Since we tend to study topics that interest us or those we are involved with, chances are we will be an insider at one point in our research careers.

Therefore, learning how to navigate some of these limitations is key. The walking meditation can prepare us for the field, so we walk into the research setting with vigilant senses. In using all five senses, we will be more open to the present moment, leading us to capture the nuance and details that we may have missed the previous times we entered into that particular context. In other words, we are using the five senses through the act of walking to reignite our beginner's mind (covered in Chapter 3) in a space that we have been countless times, which helps us see and experience everything for the very first time.

THE PRACTICE: WALKING MEDITATION

Walking meditation is a great way to bring your mindfulness into the world around you. Another benefit is that mindful walking can be practiced anytime. For example, you can practice it while you are going for a casual stroll or even as you head to school or work in the morning. The objective is to be awake and present during the walk by awakening the senses. When we are walking mindfully, we notice things we normally wouldn't because our experience becomes richer through all the senses. Sounds are sharper. Sights are more colorful. Smells are enhanced. We can stop and feel the nature around us like a leaf or hear the rustle of grass in the wind. Even taste, like the salty air, might be possible in the walking meditation. Through walking meditation, we begin to experience our body in a whole new way. All we have to do is pay attention, open ourselves to receiving the five senses and how they shape our present experience. Let's begin.

Set your timer for 15 to 20 minutes. You will begin by simply starting to walk. Bring your attention to the lower part of your body and simply notice the movement involved in walking. First, you lift your heel. Then the sole of your foot peels off the ground. Then the ball of the foot raises, and your toes follow to complete your first step. Notice how each step feels.

Feel into the balls and soles of your feet as you take each step. See if you can notice all 10 toes. Observe if you walk lightly or if there is a heaviness to each step you take. Whether your pace is fast or slow, pay close attention as each foot encounters the ground.

Now, bring your attention to how your weight shifts as you walk. See how the muscles in your legs and feet work to balance your body as you take each step.

Continue to expand your focus from your feet and legs to your body as a whole. The first thing you might notice is that your entire body moves as you walk, not just your legs. Feel how your arms move as they swing gently by your sides. Notice how your shoulders, chest, and abdomen move with your body as you walk.

If you want to, you can experiment with your pace, seeing how your body reacts when you walk fast and then when you walk slow. The slower you walk, the more sensations you are likely to notice. However, if you walk fast, you can still bring a depth of mindfulness to the experience. See if your experience varies depending on the pace of your walking.

Now, let's transition to observe tactile sensations. Notice if the surface you are walking on is hard or soft. Do you sense a cool or warm breeze in the air? Is the sun warming your body? Do you feel rain, snow, or wind against your body?

Expand your awareness to sight. Take in everything around you. Observe the people, animals, beauty of nature, houses, buildings, or any form of transportation. View all the shapes and colors of the world around you. This might be a good time to revisit the beginner's mind that we discussed in Chapter 3. Look at the world around you like you are seeing it for the first time. Soak up the sights with wonder, curiosity, and amazement.

Let's move to the sense of smell. Notice any smells around you, both strong or more subtle, pleasant or unpleasant. Focus on all of the smells around you within this moment.

Next up is sound: tuning into the sounds around you, hearing them as they arise. You may recall us learning about sound in Chapter 2 and using it to begin our mindfulness journey. Here, sound may arrive differently, since you are in motion instead of seated in a chair. Some sounds might be loud or quiet. Focus on all sounds that ebb and flow as you walk.

The last sense that we need to include in our experience is taste. Although the most difficult one to access in a walking meditation, it is still possible. For example, do you have a water bottle with you? How does the water taste? Is the sensation cold or warm? Or maybe you did not bring anything to drink; therefore, do you taste a dry mouth or sweat from the walk if it is hot out? Or maybe you taste lip balm that was previously applied or the toothpaste from your morning brushing of teeth? What tastes are you experiencing? Are they strong or weak tastes? Observe what tastes you can identify, no matter how faint.

For the last few moments, come into full sensory awareness. Tune into sights, sounds, sensations, smells, and tastes. Wake to the entire sensory experience.

As we near the end of this walking meditation, notice how you feel. What did you notice that you may have missed before? How do you feel? Do you feel relaxed, alert, and refreshed?

The walking meditation will be your practice for the next 2 weeks. Dedicate time each day to this meditation to see how this active meditation changes your senses and experiences over time. Consider changing locations every few days to see how your experiences change. Or maybe choose to walk in the opposite direction. Be open to changing your location and see how this impacts your experience. Have fun with it! Get creative with this practice since the purpose is to be active. At the end of each session, complete your *Mindful Memos*. Through this practice, you may experience changes in your senses that impact not only your ability to conduct participant observations but also enrich your senses in everyday life.

Once you have completed your 2 weeks of walking meditation, use this practice in the future before embarking on participant observation. This will be a great tool to prepare for ethnographic or case study work that includes some element of observational data. By engaging in a walking meditation prior to data collection, you will be prepared for the field by bringing awareness to all of your senses.

CONCLUSION

This chapter introduced the walking meditation as a tool for participant observation. This particular meditation is distinctive in that it includes the action of walking to develop and activate the five senses. When the senses are engaged in the research setting, participant observation data will incorporate more nuanced details that lead to rich descriptions. In turn, this leads to deeper insights about the context being studied.

KEY TAKEAWAYS

- The walking meditation is unique in that it helps us in the development of all five senses: sound, touch, sight, taste, and smell. This practice is about awakening all of the senses to prepare for the research setting.

- Participant observation is a great tool to collect primary data, especially in case study and ethnographic research where firsthand observation is desired.

- Despite the many values that accompany field work and participant observation, challenges do present themselves. A few challenges include knowing when and how to enter the field, becoming overloaded with observation data, and recognizing when insider blindness is taking over.

● The walking meditation can prepare us for the field, so we walk into the research setting with vigilant senses. In using all our senses, we will be more open to the present moment, leading us to capture the nuance and details, which cultivates thick descriptions.

● Walking meditation is a great way to bring mindfulness into the physical world around you. Another benefit is that mindful walking can be practiced anytime.

REFLECTION QUESTIONS

● What challenges might you face while conducting participant observations?

● What preconceived notions do you have about collecting data via participant observation?

● Which of your senses do you tend to privilege over the others? Why do you think you do so?

● Now that you have been practicing meditation for a few weeks, how do you feel about participating in a walking meditation? How will this experience be different for you than the meditations you have learned thus far?

THE 2-WEEK PRACTICE: WALKING MEDITATION

The walking meditation will be your meditation practice for the next 2 weeks. Dedicate time each day to complete the walking meditation to see how using all of your senses helps you develop alertness to the present moment while becoming relaxed at the same time. This unique dichotomy of the walking meditation will be key to preparing for the field and conducting participant observations. Be sure to complete the *Mindful Memos* at the end of each walking meditation. You might write down what you noticed about your senses and how you use them. Or maybe you completed a walk you do every day, but this time recognized small details that you usually miss—capture these details in your memos. Remember, the *Mindful Memos* are yours to record your experiences. The walking meditation is a great tool to enliven and bring joy to the present moment through heightened awareness using the senses.

Mindful Memos

REFERENCES

Angrosino, M., & Rosenberg, J. (2013). Observations on observation. In N. K. Denzin & Y. S. Lincoln (Eds.), *Collecting and interpreting qualitative materials* (4th ed., pp. 151–175). Sage.

DeSantis, A. D. (2002). Smoke screen: An ethnographic study of a cigar shop's collection rationalization. *Health Communication, 14*(2), 167–198. https://doi.org/10.1207/S15327027HC1402_2

Edwards, M. K., Rosenbaum, S., & Loprinzi, P. D. (2017). Differential experimental effects of a short bout of walking, meditation, or combination of walking and meditation on state anxiety among young adults. *American Journal of Health Promotion, 32*(4), 949–958. https://doi.org/10.1177/0890117717744913

Gainey, A., Himathongkam, T., Tanaka, H., & Suksom, D. (2016). Effects of Buddhist walking meditation on glycemic control and vascular function in patients with type 2 diabetes. *Complementary Therapies in Medicine, 26*, 92–97. https://doi.org/10.1016/j.ctim.2016.03.009

Kim, S., & Ki, J. (2014). A case study on the effects of the creative art therapy with stretching and walking meditation—Focusing on the improvement of emotional expression and alleviation of somatisation symptoms in a neurasthenic adolescent. *The Arts in Psychotherapy, 41*(1), 71–78. https://doi.org/10.1016/j.aip.2013.11.002

Merriam, S. B., & Tisdell, E. J. (2016). *Qualitative research: A guide to design and implementation* (4th ed.). Jossey-Bass.

Patton, M. Q. (2015). *Qualitative research and evaluation methods* (4th ed.). Sage.

Taylor, J. (2011). The intimate insider: Negotiating the ethics of friendship when doing insider research. *Qualitative Research, 11*(3), 3–22.

Tracy, S. J. (2020). *Qualitative research methods: Collecting evidence, crafting analysis, communicating impact* (2nd ed.). Wiley-Blackwell.

Yin, R. K. (2018). *Case study research: Design and methods* (6th ed.). Sage.

6 NOTING TO DEAL WITH DATA MANAGEMENT

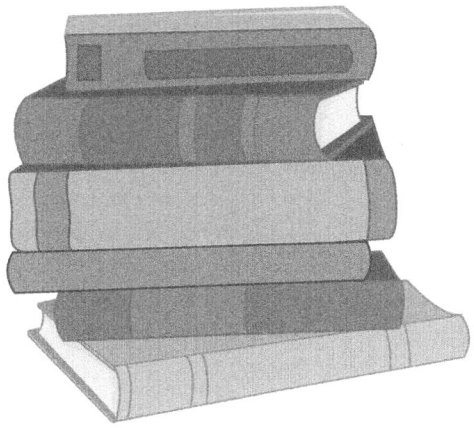

The sixth chapter, Noting to Deal With Data Management, addresses data management and how to remain organized in the research process. You will find this chapter is one of the most comprehensive in terms of applicable suggestions. But don't be concerned; you won't lose the sense of curiosity and playfulness you had been developing in the preceding chapters of this book. The noting meditation that is discussed in this chapter is actually one of the more abstract meditations, and this helps balance the structured suggestions for dealing with data management. The steps for a noting meditation are included to cultivate new space in the mind, which builds on the previous practices in the book. At the end of the chapter, a conclusion, key takeaways, and reflection questions are included. A space for the *Mindful Memos* is also available, along with a summary of the practice.

USING THE PRACTICE OF NOTING TO RIDE THE WAVE

Let's explore the practice of noting. This technique can be helpful because we have all had research experiences, especially when dealing with data management, where we've gotten caught up in the data, and it isn't until we sit down and begin analysis that realize we are a bit lost. In other words, all we see are data, unable to take in the bigger picture. When we feel lost in the research process, we might develop feelings of doubt, worry, and confusion, or experience emotions of being unsure, indecisive, or frustrated. Even the most experienced scholars have overwhelming moments during a research project. On the opposite end of emotions, we might sense excitement and elation about the insights we've discovered. These experiences can create tunnel vision as we go looking for the same findings in other data sources. The noting technique can be a useful skill to develop so we are not swept by these thoughts and emotions that often stem from working with data.

Ultimately, the noting practice is about creating space by acknowledging the feelings and emotions we have and then letting them pass. When we try to run or hide from emotions, they often sweep us under like a giant wave crashing down on us. If you have ever boogie boarded or bodysurfed in the ocean, you know you must ride the wave's crest, its face, not its trough. If you try to swim away from the wave or push against it, the wave will ultimately crash down on you. However, if you simply ride with the wave, you will gently wash ashore. The noting meditation is how we ride or navigate through the waves or our emotions and feelings.

The Noting Meditation Functions.   Noting has two important functions. First, it keeps us present. We are less likely to wander off when we are constantly noting our experience. Like the breath, the practice serves as an anchor to the present moment. Second, labeling our thoughts and experiences helps us identify what is going on in the mind. For example, we might not realize we are constantly planning until the thought continues to present itself during our practice. Or we don't realize that we are frustrated with our research process until the feeling continues to appear. Only then can we begin to do something about the planning or the frustration. The more mindful we are about our thoughts and emotions, the more we are able to address those thoughts and emotions that continue to exist in the mind.

Research on the Noting Meditation.   The mind is an organ that controls our muscles, and for it to work at its optimum capacity, it needs to be exercised and trained. The heart works in the same fashion—it is an organ that needs exercise to become stronger. The noting practice is one of the many meditation techniques you are learning in this book, and the medical community has investigated its benefits. For example, Whitfield-Gabrieli et al. (2017) found that patients with schizophrenia who participated in the noting practice over time were able to change how they perceived internal thoughts and feelings from external stimuli. Another study looked at physician burnout and the potential results of participating in the noting practice over time (Roy et al., 2020). The findings indicated that after practicing noting for 3 months, the physician participants experienced less burnout and anxiety related to their jobs (Roy et al. 2020). These insights demonstrate the value of engaging with the noting meditation.

BECOMING AN ORGANIZED RESEARCHER

Being organized is a crucial part of the research process. In qualitative work, the audit trail is often used as one of the tools for organization, which ensures the credibility of the research. An audit trail helps readers follow the researcher's decisions throughout the process, by detailing "how data were collected, how categories were derived, and how decisions were made throughout the inquiry" (Merriam & Tisdell, 2016, p. 252). Richards (2015) explains that quality research comes from "the researcher's ability to show convincingly how they got there, and how they built confidence that this was the best account possible. This is why qualitative research has a special need for project history, and in the form of a diary or log of processes" (p. 143). Your diary or log becomes the place in which you record your processes and ultimately serves as your audit trail.

GETTING ORGANIZED

To get organized for the research process might mean we need to organize other parts of our lives. Take a look around you and make an inventory of what might need attention. Does your pantry need to be cleaned out? Is your fridge full of expired items? Maybe you have a closet with items that need to be donated. Or is it finally time to clean out your email inbox? As you examine your surroundings, consider where you can get organized to create space.

Although the audit trail implies structure and rigidity, know that you have the flexibility and freedom to make it work for you. For example, to document your data collection and analysis, you may decide to use colorful markers in a spiralbound notebook or the voice memo app in your phone. Or possibly, your research team meets over coffee to discuss the progress of your project, and you find capturing your audit trail on drink napkins makes the most sense. It is not the way in which you capture the information that matters—what matters is that you are logging the details of the research process so that you can explain it clearly and comprehensively to your readers. This is how professional researchers and academic scholars demonstrate excellent credibility and rigor.

POTENTIAL DATA MANAGEMENT CHALLENGES

Much of my research process is defined by being organized. I have colleagues who prefer to be more "creative" throughout their research process in terms of organization and steps, but I personally choose to have a strategic approach when it comes to managing data. This does not mean I am not open to the fluid nature of the qualitative research process, but instead, my personal approach is underpinned by organization, so I am very confident about the data collected and, in turn, analyzed. My organizational process is a way to ensure rigor and allows me to be transparent with my readers about the steps I took to arrive at the insights answering the research question(s).

As we discuss data management issues, I will be including my own processes for how I remain organized in addition to how the noting practice can help navigate the copious amount of data that emerges from a qualitative research project. But remember, these are just descriptions of what works for me. As you read, be thinking about what works best for you or how you might adapt your approach in a way that will help you in the analysis and writing phases of your project. The goal is to find a meaningful organizational process while using the noting practice to create space in the midst of data without sacrificing rigor.

Transcribing and Getting Your Data Ready. Before we cover data management, we need to discuss the process of transcription since that is how data develop. With advancements in technology, this process has drastically improved; most virtual meeting software like Zoom and Microsoft Teams can create a transcript of the audio recorded session. In addition, platforms such as Otter.ai and Fireflies.ai provide AI-generated transcripts. It was only a few years ago that most qualitative researchers spent hours transcribing one interview or focus group.

Nevertheless, you cannot take these AI-generated transcripts as accurate and ready to go for data management. The transcripts must be checked for accuracy before data analysis can even begin (which will be covered in the next chapter). The best way to ensure the transcripts are accurate is to listen to the audio from the focus group or interview while reading the transcript. When errors are identified, you will be able to correct them in real time. In addition, if the AI did not catch utterances such as "ah" and "um," these can be added to confirm the transcripts are verbatim.

As you might know or can imagine, this process is incredibly time-consuming and tedious. I have even had graduate students comment that the checking for accuracy of AI-generated transcripts has led them to rethink whether to transcribe their own data in the future—they thought it just might be easier to transcribe the data themselves. However, the noting practice can be helpful in working through this laborious and sometimes monotonous process of checking transcripts from outside sources. Specifically, pausing to pay attention to the thoughts and feelings regarding the experience can be very helpful. You might feel bored, uninterested, distracted, excited, or indifferent to the process. However, the most important part is the intentional pause to check-in and see how you are feeling and what you are thinking. The noting becomes the anchor to the present moment, which can be a great tool when we are working on a tedious task, like checking transcripts, that may result in us getting preoccupied or sidetracked.

Organizational Issues and Paving Your Own Way. The main issue you may run into with managing data is how to keep everything organized. Carelessly saving audio or transcript files or scribbling notes down in different places will quickly lead to a sense of being overwhelmed when it comes time to begin analyzing data. You will most likely find yourself asking: Where did I put that audio file? Or you might spend hours looking for participant observation notes. This process robs you of mental effort that needs to be reserved for collecting more data or analyzing the data you have. If the process is not organized, energy will be expended and progress impeded.

My organizational process comes down to very minute details. For example, I take jottings or field notes in one specific spiraled notebook dedicated to each new research project. Also, all electronic files are labeled and filed in a way that ensures easy retrieval but also straightforward identification of which participant the file is associated with from the study.

One of my most important organizational tools is what I refer to as my "Sample Spreadsheet." I create a spreadsheet for my sample that is used throughout the research project. The column headers may change depending on the study, but the purpose is to capture details about the participants, communication exchanges, memos, transcript pages, and interview length. For example, I might include the organization a person works for, tenure at the organization, title, type of organization, and where they are located. The memos are my initial thoughts and insights immediately following an interview. Usually, this information comes from the jottings I write while having the conversation. A column for follow-up and member checks is also included. I immediately include the interview time and later add in the number of transcript pages. All this information ensures I am capturing the correct details about my participants along the way, which is a portion of the audit trail, and it helps me write the method section of the final paper.

The noting practice can also be a tool to navigate organizational issues. Given how data can quickly add up in a qualitative research study, we might have feelings, emotions, and/or thoughts regarding the data management process. We might feel inspired, confused, elated, overwhelmed, happy, indifferent, or even frustrated. Often, it isn't until we take a break and spend time specifically exploring how we think and feel about the data we are collecting and the process we are using that we begin to identify our experiences regarding data management. When we shed light on these thoughts and feelings, we are able to let them pass so they don't bog us down, and we can continue on with the present research study.

THE PRACTICE: NOTING MEDITATION

The noting meditation is a bit more abstract than some of the practices we have explored thus far because the practice requires you to wait until your mind presents a feeling or emotion. This is different than the body scan or walking meditation where we are actively searching for items to anchor us to the present moment. However, this particular meditation is preparing us for the open awareness practice that will come in the next chapter, which is the culmination of the meditation practices.

The idea behind the noting technique is it helps us stay present and not get carried away by our thoughts and emotions. The way the technique works is when we experience a thought or emotion during a meditation, we calmly note it instead of getting lost, carried away, or distracted by it. The act of noting a thought or emotion is like whispering "ah-ha" in the mind.

The first step of the practice is noting emotions and thoughts with one-word labels as they arise. For example, to label an emotion as it appears, you might say to yourself "happy" or "sad" or "excited" or "calm" or "confused" or "distracted." Or you might begin to notice what your thoughts are doing and label them as such. For example, "wanting" or "hoping" or "striving" or "ruminating" or "planning" might be labels that you use. By rehearsing giving our thoughts and emotions a one-word label throughout the noting practice, we can acknowledge what is happening in the present moment but should refrain from getting swept away by our thoughts.

The second step is to keep repeating the same label or word until you notice the thought or emotion has dissipated to the extent that it is no longer active. For example, you will say in your mind "planning . . . planning . . . planning . . . planning" until your planning thought has moved to the background of your mind. The goal is to not minimize our thoughts or get swept away by them. We just want to view them as visitors, and then show them to the exit.

Let's begin. Set your timer for 15 to 20 minutes. Find a comfortable seat, in a quiet place where you can remain focused, yet relaxed. Take a moment to settle into the space, resting your hands gently in your lap or down at your sides. Feel the seat beneath you. Take a deep breath and close your eyes. Relax any tension in the face, softening your eyes and forehead. Use this moment to tune inward, into your breath. Take a few deep breaths. Begin with a long inhale followed by a long, audible exhale. Repeat these deep breaths three to five more times. As you exhale, being to notice places in your body where you could relax. Maybe you need to release the tension in your shoulders or in your face. Release the gripping of your hands or the tightness in your back. Then, gently release the breath into a simple breathing pattern that is natural and easy.

Bring your awareness to the breath. Take natural breaths, where the breath is the anchor to the present moment. Become aware of how the breath comes into the body and then how it leaves the body. Follow the natural breath as it comes in and out. Notice the small pause that happens at the end of the exhale and then again at the top of the inhale.

Now that you are grounded in the present moment, let's begin the practice of noting. Anytime a thought or emotion arises, silently note it. You can note a feeling as excited or calm or any emotion that comes to mind. Or you might have thoughts about anything from worrying to planning to ruminating. You might begin to think that it is odd that you don't have as many thoughts as you should. However, the goal is not to go looking for thoughts but becoming aware of them as they emerge. Feel free to follow the breath as an anchor to center you while waiting for thoughts and feelings to surface during this meditation.

As thoughts and emotions appear, try not to label them with a value such as good or bad. You may recall that in Chapter 3 we discussed the problem with labeling. Labeling your experience during a meditation practice or anything in the research process with a quantifier can be limiting. This remains the same with the noting practice. Therefore, avoid labeling a thought or emotion as good or bad, and instead, treat all of them equally. Be sure to avoid getting drawn into the content around the thought or emotion. Just note it as a simple observation. You will find that the thought or emotion will, in fact, pass. In between thoughts and emotions, the breath remains your mainstay to the present moment.

Once the timer goes off, take a few deep breaths, relaxing into this present state while holding space for all emotions and thoughts that have come to the surface during your experience. Exercise gratitude for your effort of working with your experience in this mindful way. Bring your attention back to the room. Wiggle your fingers and toes. And when you are ready, slowly open your eyes.

You may have felt some of this practice was challenging at times, but sticking with it and not getting caught in the narratives or the stories surrounding the thoughts or emotions gives you a skillset that can translate into a rich research process. This will be your practice for the next 2 weeks. Spending time working with the noting practice in the coming weeks, you will get a sense of how this meditation can benefit you and your ability to manage data.

Be sure to complete your *Mindful Memos* after each session. It will be especially important to capture what feelings and emotions consistently arise over the next 2 weeks. In acknowledging the thoughts and emotions that present themselves, you will be able to work through them in a way that creates space. Creating space is incredibly helpful in the research process, especially when we start to feel overwhelmed with data. As we create space in our surroundings and in our minds, we are more open to the amounts of data we collect in the research process. The organizational piece also helps ensure the quality of data we are analyzing to answer our research questions. This will ultimately set the stage for the next chapter, which addresses data analysis.

This practice can be used in conjunction with the other components we have discussed regarding data collection. I personally revisit the noting meditation regularly and use it as a personal check to see how I am feeling. Anytime you are feeling overwhelmed or inundated with data, return to the noting practice. This practice will help you acknowledge the feelings and emotions you have in the data management process, allowing them to pass.

CONCLUSION

This chapter introduced the noting meditation and how it could be used with data management and the subsequent thoughts and feelings associated with the amount of data a qualitative project usually encompasses. It included information about the noting meditation in regard to its psychological benefits and implications for the research process. A section of the chapter was dedicated to improving organizational research processes and presented my approaches for staying organized. The noting meditation directions were included, as well as a description of how this practice can be used to navigate whatever thoughts and feelings present themselves during the research activity. This practice is ideal to revisit at any time since it helps us get in-tune with what we are thinking and feeling.

KEY TAKEAWAYS

- This chapter explored the practice of noting. The noting meditation can be a useful skill to develop so we are not swept by thoughts and emotions that often stem from working with data.

- Being organized is a crucial part of the research process. In qualitative work, the audit trail is often used as one of the tools for organization, which ensures the credibility of the research.

- The practical aspects presented in this chapter encourage you to uncover and solidify the ways in which you can remain organized throughout the research process. I shared my own; now it is time to discover your approach.

- The noting meditation was introduced, which helps us stay present, not getting carried away by our thoughts and emotions. The way the technique works is when we experience a thought or emotion during a meditation, we calmly note it instead of getting lost, carried away, or distracted.

REFLECTION QUESTIONS

- How would you rate your research organization strategies at this point? What could you do to improve how you remain organized throughout the research process?

- Do you feel as though being organized stifles your creative process? Why or why not?

- After your first noting meditation, what emotions or thoughts surprised you? How do you feel after acknowledging them and then letting them pass?

THE 2-WEEK PRACTICE: NOTING MEDITATION

The noting meditation will be your practice for the next 2 weeks. Be sure to dedicate time each day to engage with the noting meditation so you can work on riding through your thoughts and emotions. Although this practice is presented as a tool for dealing with data management, you will find the noting meditation helpful at many points in the research process. I would encourage you to continue this practice again alongside the others presented in this book. The *Mindful Memos* will be a crucial tool to rely on to recognize the repeated feelings and emotions you might have, so you can let them go. Be open to any and all of the feelings and emotions you are experiencing. May you enjoy the benefit of riding the waves of emotions and feelings to land on the shore of newly found space.

Mindful Memos

_____

_____

_____

_____

_____

_____

_____

_____

_____

_____

_____

_____

_____

_____

_____

_____

_____

_____

_____

_____

_____

_____

_____

_____

REFERENCES

Merriam, S. B., & Tisdell, E. J. (2016). *Qualitative research: A guide to design and implementation* (4th ed.). Jossey-Bass.

Richards, L. (2015). *Handling qualitative data.* (3rd ed.). Sage.

Roy, A., Druker, S., Hoge, E., & Brewer, J. (2020). Physician anxiety and burnout: Symptom correlates and a prospective pilot study of app-delivered mindfulness training. *JMIR Mhealth Uhealth, 8*(4), 15608.

Whitfield-Gabrieli, S., Bauer, C., Okano, K., Nestor, P., Del Re, E., Gosh, S., & Niznikiewicz, M. (2017). M64. Real time fMRI feedback targeting default mode network (DMN) reduces auditory hallucinations. *Schizophrenia Bulletin, 43*(1), S233. https://doi.org/10.1093/schbul/sbx022.059

7 EXERCISING OPEN AWARENESS IN DATA ANALYSIS

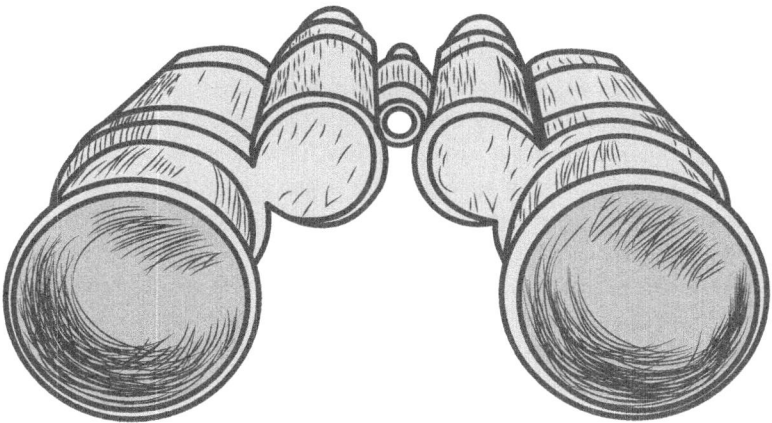

The seventh chapter, Exercising Open Awareness in Data Analysis, begins by introducing the open awareness practice, then previews the basic approaches to data analysis, and transitions to discuss the potential challenges a researcher will have to circumvent when conducting data analysis and how an open awareness practice can assist in addressing such challenges. Instructions for the open awareness meditation are included. A conclusion, key takeaways, and reflection questions complete the chapter. A space for the *Mindful Memos* is included, along with a summary of the practice.

OPEN AWARENESS

The open awareness meditation is about expanding the mind and combines many of the preceding practices we have explored in this book. Specifically, this practice includes different stages that move from the breath to sounds to the body to thoughts and feelings and finally to whatever might materialize in the present moment. Because of the transition from one practice to the next, it requires a more skilled practitioner, which is why this training is found in the latter part of this book.

You will want to think of sitting in open awareness as welcoming every part of your experience in the present moment. Sometimes the focus will be on the breath. Sounds will be the anchor in the next part of the meditation, followed by time focusing on the body. This will be concluded by thoughts and feelings. The outcome will be to welcome all of these experiences as they ebb and flow, moving from the forefront to the background during the meditation.

There might be moments when you focus on your breath, but in the next second, you might feel a sensation in your knee, which could be followed by a thought about your next meal. Also, consider moments when you will just be present, waiting for the next sensation to present itself. The absence of any feeling, thought, or sensation is another way in which we attune to the present moment. Although this may sound like a lot more effort, it actually isn't. Instead, it's simply about exercising an effortless presence. The idea is to sit with an intentional, nonjudgmental openness of everything you are experiencing in the meditation.

As with many of the other practices in this book, researchers have investigated the physiological benefits of the open awareness practice. Understanding the practices *actually* change the ways in which our brains function is important to understanding the benefits. For example, Oishi et al. (2021) conducted a study with 41 novice meditators, where they engaged in a 30-minute open awareness meditation and then participated in subsequent testing. The authors found that following an open awareness meditation, participants reduced their cortisol levels, which means they were able to reduce stress (Oishi et al., 2021). In addition, Cullen et al. (2021) discovered that following a long-term meditation practice over 20 weeks, participants experienced a decrease in stress, anxiety, and depression at multiple points throughout the treatment. Furthermore, Baad et al. (2019) found that those who participated in the open awareness meditation experienced greater creativity in idea generation.

Developing Open Awareness in Data Analysis. Given its purpose of expansion and heightened awareness of the present moment, the open awareness meditation is the ideal fit for data analysis. This particular meditation requires an openness in the meditator, welcoming everything that presents itself at one moment in time. We may move from sounds to a body sensation to a thought and back to the breath. Here, we are accepting whatever may arise while we are in our active meditation. During data analysis, we need to be active, alert, and open to whatever emerges from the data. In addition, there needs to be an awareness of blind spots. Blind spots could be only looking for certain codes, privileging one data point over another, or relying on what previous literature says. These areas of preference and others are often the results of the mind operating on autopilot, where we aren't paying close attention to how our previous knowledge and experience are limiting the ways in which we analyze the data.

APPROACHES TO DATA ANALYSIS

Analyzing qualitive data is a complex process that requires a sharpened level of thinking and awareness. Merriam and Tisdell (2016) discuss that the quickest way to undermine your data is to conduct a sloppy analysis. The ultimate goal should be to make sense out of the data in a way that answers your research question(s) (Merriam & Tisdell, 2016).

Many of the qualitative approaches provide detailed steps regarding how data should be analyzed. For example, Strauss and Corbin (1998) offered steps for data analysis in a grounded theory study, where the focus is on the constant comparative method. The constant comparative method organizes and categories data into groups that are then compared and contrasted with the goal of developing a new theory. Moustakas (1994) provided the data analysis procedures for a phenomenological study, which relies on the hermeneutical approach to arrive at the essence of the phenomenon. Both approaches are inductive in nature and allow the researcher to be open to the themes that emerge from the data. To the contrary, Miles et al. (2014) take a more deductive approach by encouraging the researcher to develop a codebook with defined codes prior to beginning data analysis. Tracy (2020) takes a combined approach, calling it "phronetic iterative analysis" (p. 208). Here, the goal is to move back and forth between the emergent nature of the data and existing theories and explanations to create robust findings from the data. This iterative approach helps the researcher move away from descriptive, surface-level insights. I encourage you to explore the original cites listed here or others to discover and learn about the best approach for analyzing your data.

One final note—transparency in reporting the data analysis steps is imperative. The reader cannot trust the findings if the steps to analyzing data are vague and unclear. When I review qualitative research papers for journals, I provide considerable feedback asking the author(s) to be more detailed in their analysis procedures. This means I am not looking for one particular way for the data to be analyzed—I simply want the details so I can understand how the authors arrived at their findings. The clearer we are as researchers in our method sections, the more the reviewers—and, in turn, readers—can understand and trust our insights. Providing robust data analysis details also has the broader implication of shifting negative connotations of the methods in spaces where qualitative data analysis is still assumed to be less than its quantitative counterpart.

POTENTIAL DATA ANALYSIS CHALLENGES

Bottom line: Qualitative data analysis is hard work. It does not matter if you take an inductive or deductive approach with a defined codebook, or choose to code by hand with several colored highlighters, or use computer data analysis software; the process of analyzing qualitative data is tedious and mentally challenging. Because of this, you will want to analyze data when you are functioning at your best. If you do your finest work in the middle of the night, then that is when you should analyze data. Or if you are like me and work best first thing in the morning, then accommodate this for your optimum analysis. Create an environment where you can remain focused and comfortable with minimal distractions for a period of time. This will set you up for success in terms of analysis.

In addition, the open awareness meditation can be incorporated as part of your data analysis rituals to prepare your mind for the data. When engaging in the open awareness meditation, you will be able to use it to overcome some of the challenges that qualitative researchers face in the data analysis process. These include getting started, remaining focused, and building themes or arriving at nondescriptive conclusions. Remember, this list is not exhaustive, and you will encounter your own, unique challenges. In any case, you can rely on the open awareness meditation as a guiding light to work through your data analysis stumbling blocks.

Getting Started. One of the hardest parts of data analysis is simply getting started. When I work with graduate students, they often struggle with beginning the data analysis process, which in most cases is some version of open coding. Open coding is defined as highlighting or identifying any portion of the data that might be useful (Merriam & Tisdell, 2016). In other words, you are allowing yourself to be open to anything that emerges from the data (Merriam & Tisdell, 2016). Tracy (2020) suggests that coding is "the active process of identifying data as belonging to, or representing, some type of phenomenon. This phenomenon may be a concept, belief, action, theme, cultural practice, or relationship" (p. 213). She refers to open coding as "primary-cycle coding" or the first round of coding (p. 219). Ultimately, coding is about making sense of the data in a way that we can begin to answer our research questions beyond a descriptive nature. However, coding can oftentimes be an intimidating process to begin.

Take, for example, a former student of mine, Tory (her name has been changed here). She has many years of experience in the context in which she is conducting interviews. As an insider, she has collected incredibly rich data and made her participants feel comfortable in the research process. Interview skills oftentimes take time to develop, but she is a natural. I have enjoyed reading her transcripts and witnessing her conversational approach. It is now time for her to begin data analysis, but she is having trouble getting started. She has conducted several interviews, but her project is at a stalemate because she cannot get over the open coding hump. We have discussed her experiences and where she is in her research process. I tell her she just needs to start and not to be concerned with a "right or wrong" experience. She simply needs to take the risk and begin to wade around in the data. Although it can often feel like wading through mud, seeing this experience like a child playing in mud for the first time can help us shift our perceptions. Kids have no limitations when splashing in a mud puddle; they are exploring and welcoming in the totality of the experience.

For most novice researchers, open or primary-cycle coding feels like jumping into the ocean for the first time and forgetting how to swim. The vastness of the ocean supersedes the muscle memory of an experienced swimmer. Similarly, opening a transcript or field notes to analyze causes the researcher's mind to go blank even though they have read about and practiced the skills needed to begin the coding process.

The open awareness meditation and its ability to ground you to the present moment is a helpful tool to navigate these inhibiting feelings and thoughts that might surface and prevent you from getting started. When we engage in the open awareness meditation, we are able to unhook from repetitive and limiting thoughts. The practice allows us to center our minds and clear space to focus on the task at hand without getting distracted by thoughts that tell us we must do it perfectly.

Remaining Focused. As mentioned earlier, analyzing qualitative data is time-consuming and can be mentally exhausting. Not only do you have to create an environment that sets you up for success, but you also need the mental capacity to remain focused for indefinite periods of time.

Let's talk about the environment first. What do you require to remain comfortable and focused? Do you need the temperature to be warm or cold? How about your chair? Do you prefer the couch, a chaise lounge, or a traditional desk chair? Do you have special preferences for lighting, like bright, natural light, or dimmed house lights? Do you like to have snacks with you? If so, what kinds of snacks? I once saw a post on Twitter that asked followers for the best snacks to eat while analyzing qualitative data since most of us are working with a computer or papers that can't get dirty. People suggested pretzels, carrots, raisins, grapes, celery with peanut butter, and chocolate-covered nuts as examples. Things to avoid were those that made your fingers dirty, like seasoned chips or cheesy popcorn. Or maybe you should consider your beverages; do you want coffee or tea, along with water? I would encourage you to spend a few moments to jot down your needs for the environment so you can operate at your highest level.

Ultimately, you need to create the optimum environment to analyze data. As you mentally note what you need to be successful, be sure to save time for participating in the open awareness meditation. This meditation should be done before you begin data analysis so that your mind is alert and open to whatever presents itself while you analyze data.

Remaining focused also means you need to know when to leave analysis for another day. Trying to analyze all your data in a single day is impossible and would completely undermine the work you did to collect quality data. This means that you will need to be aware of your personal limitations for the amount of data you can analyze in one sitting. The open awareness meditation can also be a helpful tool in recognizing when it is time to call it quits. This practice allows us to tune completely into our current experiences and heightens our awareness of everything we are experiencing in that moment— which, in this case, could mean mental exhaustion or physical fatigue. In both cases, recognize signs to end data analysis for the day and return the following day to start again with a fresh mind.

Developing Themes. One of the key aspects of qualitative data analysis is to work toward theme development. This is the stage of data analysis when repetitive codes are collapsed together or codes that are not relevant to the research question(s) are removed. We also need to look at our data through fresh eyes to make sure we have not missed anything or had blinders on regarding one particular theme, and therefore missed important nuances. In addition, this is the stage when we need to ask ourselves, "What is the story the data are telling me?"

We have an intimate connection with our data since we collected them, transcribed them, and/or checked them for accuracy, and now we are pouring over the data to understand them in a way that answers our research question(s). We might struggle with seeing the bigger picture of how the tens of hundreds of codes we assigned can work together to tell a meaningful story that adequately represents the lived experiences of our participants, but that is the goal of qualitative data analysis. Detailing the participants' experiences is the emic approach, or the perspective from the inside (Merriam & Tisdell, 2016). Simultaneously, our findings need to incorporate an etic perspective, which brings outside information, like existing theories and/or scholarship, to make sense of the data (Merriam & Tisdell, 2016). By using the etic perspective, our study will most likely have a contribution to theory development in our respective field. The balancing act between the etic and emic aligns with Tracy's (2020) approach to analysis.

To get to theme development, we must be open to what our data are saying and have a willingness to see things from different vantage points. In phenomenology, this is called imaginative variation, where the goal is to ask questions of the data so that nuance can be revealed (Moustakas, 1994). However, researchers hit stumbling blocks when they begin to see their data in linear fashion versus contextual (Merriam & Tisdell, 2016), where the focus is looking at data from different angles.

The open awareness meditation can strengthen our ability to see data from multiple vantage points to work toward theme development. Just how the practice teaches us to welcome in a myriad of experiences in the present moment, this same level of openness and curiosity can be applied to data analysis. The open awareness meditation strengthens our ability to be open to the entirety of our experiences by focusing on the breath, sound, the body, thoughts, and feelings. We are acutely attuned to the present moment in a way that we can closely catch all that is occurring. This same attention can strengthen our ability in data analysis so that we can uncover the nuance or seek imaginative variation. When we begin to probe below the surface, we start to see the implications of the data and the deeper meaning of our research.

THE PRACTICE: OPEN AWARENESS MEDITATION

The open awareness meditation is one that combines many of the practices we have explored in previous chapters. Specifically, we will begin with focusing on the breath, as we always do. Next, the focus will be on sounds, followed by a short body scan. Then, we will appraise our thoughts and feelings as they emerge, which we discussed in the last chapter. Finally, we will sit in open awareness, welcoming in whatever presents itself, using our *entire* experience to anchor us to the present moment. At one moment, it might be sounds that transport us to the present, and the next moment it might be a thought conveying an intimate understanding. Sit with whatever presents itself during our 20 to 25 minute meditation, our longest yet.

Start by finding a quiet place to sit and setting your alarm for 20 to 25 minutes. Remember, we want to find a place where we can sit in the quiet, with a straight back so we can remain alert, yet relaxed. Close your eyes and place your hands in your lap or comfortably on your knees. Relax your neck and shoulders. Feel your body settle into the comfortable, seated posture. And as you begin to settle into your space, turn to the breath. A calming breath, a breath that builds a connection between your mind and body. Notice how it draws into your body and how it leaves the body. Notice how you don't have to try to breathe, that it occurs naturally, with minimal effort.

Use the breath to transition from where you just were to the present moment by taking long, deep inhales and long, slow exhales.

After you have spent a few moments focusing on the breath, begin to expand your awareness to your body, paying attention to its entirety. You are now using the body to ground within the present moment. Focus your attention on each part of the body. Start by bringing your attention to the top of your head and scalp, feeling whatever is happening in this area. Continue to move throughout the body from the top of your head to your face to your shoulders, arms, and then the hands and fingers. What do you feel as you move throughout each part of your body? Next, move your focus to your chest, back, and stomach, continuing to the legs and finally to the feet and toes. If you feel any tension throughout, gently relax by using the breath to help the rigidity soften.

Now, let us transition the practice to listening to sounds as our hook to the present. Begin by noticing in this moment the sounds in the room. What do you hear? Do you hear a sound in your immediate space? Are you able to hear sounds that are far away? As you focus on sounds, be sure not to get lost in thinking about the sounds or focusing on what is making the sound or even labeling the sound. Just rest in the experience of listening, without judging or identifying the sound. You might hear sounds from the body, from the room you are in, or from nature outside. There might also be times when there are no sounds, and in these cases, focus on the silence. You have nothing to do, nothing to fix or change about this moment, but accept it exactly as it is.

Let us spread our awareness to the thoughts and emotions that we might be experiencing in the moment. Anytime a thought or emotion arises, silently recognize it. You can note a thought as any emotion that comes to mind. The goal is not to investigate your thoughts but simply to become aware of them. When they arise, acknowledge them, and then let them pass. See your thoughts and feelings as clouds passing above you. Try not to get caught up in the story behind them—simply let them pass.

The last stage of the open awareness meditation is to sit and be present with whatever might arise. You could hear a sound that brings you into the present moment. Or you could use the body sensations you experience to heighten your awareness. But it might be passing thoughts and feelings that increase your presence, or it might be a combination of the above. However, what is most important is that you sit with everything you are experiencing in the present moment—this is open awareness. It is a skill we have been working toward in each of our chapters, and one that takes time to cultivate. If you ever get lost in your experience, know that you can always come back to the breath. Try to simply be open to whatever manifests in your present moment.

As the meditation comes to a close, take a few long, deep breaths, allowing yourself to come back into the room. Flex and loosen your fingers and toes. Inhale gratitude toward yourself for taking this time to be present and exhale the relaxed feelings you have cultivated through the open awareness meditation. When you are ready, gently open your eyes.

The open awareness meditation is your daily practice for the next 2 weeks. Dedicate time each day for 20 to 25 minutes to engage in the practice. Following the practice, be sure to complete your *Mindful Memos*. Write down your thoughts, feelings, and sensations along with anything you notice about your experience. As always, these entries are the way in which we can witness the change that occurs from our meditation practice.

Know you can return to the open awareness practice anytime you feel the need to expand your awareness. It will be especially important to revisit this particular practice before you sit down to analyze data. Make the open awareness meditation part of your data analysis ritual, where you use it to clear your mind to magnify your awareness to the extent that it allows you to see data with fresh eyes. It is also the ideal tool anytime you are feeling stuck with the analysis process. Sitting in open awareness sharpens our minds in a way so we aren't just operating on autopilot as we analyze data. This enhances the quality of our findings and contribution to the success of the project.

CONCLUSION

This chapter introduced the open awareness meditation and how it could be applied to data analysis. Specifically, the chapter covered how the open awareness meditation is practiced, and its benefits to the research process. The open awareness meditation can be a great tool for researchers to use when they are having problems getting started, remaining focused, or developing deeper insights or themes from the coded data. The chapter also included the directions to participate in the open awareness meditation.

KEY TAKEAWAYS

- The open awareness meditation is about expanding the mind and combines many of the practices we have explored in this book. Specifically, the practice allows the meditator to move from the breath to sounds to the body to thoughts and feelings and finally to whatever might suddenly be in the present moment.

- The process of analyzing qualitative data is tedious and mentally exhausting, which means you will want to analyze data when you are functioning at your best.

- The open awareness meditation can prepare your mind for data analysis.

- When engaging in the open awareness meditation, you will be able to use it to overcome some of the challenges that qualitative researchers face in the data analysis process. These include getting started, remaining focused, and building themes or arriving at nondescriptive conclusions.

REFLECTION QUESTIONS

- What intimidates you about analyzing data?

- Do you gravitate toward an inductive approach or deductive approach for data analysis? Why is this your preference?

- How do you think it will feel to sit in open awareness, where you welcome whatever comes up for you during the experience?

- What challenges might you face while sitting in open awareness? How will you work through these challenges?

- Given that this is our longest meditation practice so far, how does this make you feel?

THE 2-WEEK PRACTICE: OPEN AWARENESS MEDITATION

The open awareness meditation is your practice for the next 2 weeks. Use this practice as a way to open your mind and mentally prepare for data analysis, dedicating time each day to the practice. Remember, qualitative data analysis requires a lot of us mentally, so having a tool to relax the mind while sharpening awareness will enhance how you analyze your data. Ensure that you also make time to complete the *Mindful Memos* following each session. Because analyzing qualitative data requires a significant amount of gray matter from your brain, use this unique practice to restore and replenish what has been expended.

Mindful Memos

REFERENCES

Baas, M., Nevicka, B., & Ten Velden, F. S. (2021). When paying attention pays off: The mindfulness skill act with awareness promotes creative idea generation in groups. *European Journal of Work and Organizational Psychology, 29*, 619–632. http s://doi.org/10.1080/1359432X.2020.1727889

Cullen, B., Eichel, K., Lindahl, J. R., Rahrig, H., Kini, N., Flahive, J., & Britton, W. B. (2021). The contributions of focused attention and open monitoring in mindfulness-based cognitive therapy for affective disturbances: A 3-armed randomized dismantling trial. *PLOS ONE, 16*, e0244838. https://doi.org/10.1371/j ournal.pone.0244838

Merriam, S. B., & Tisdell, E. J. (2016). *Qualitative research: A guide to design and implementation* (4th ed.). Jossey-Bass.

Miles, M. B., Huberman, A. M., & Saldaña, J. (2014). *Qualitative data analysis: A methods sourcebook* (3rd ed.). Sage.

Moustakas, C. E. (1994). *Phenomenological research methods.* Sage.

Ooishi, Y., Fujino, M., Inoue, V., Nomura, M., & Kitagawa, N. (2021). Differential effects of focused attention and open monitoring meditation on autonomic cardiac modulation and cortisol secretion. *Frontiers in Physiology, 12*, 675899. https://doi.org/10.3389/fphys.2021.675899

Strauss, A. L., & Corbin, J. M. (1998). *Basics of qualitative research: Techniques and procedures for developing grounded theory* (2nd ed.). Sage.

Tracy, S. J. (2020). *Qualitative research methods: Collecting evidence, crafting analysis, communicating impact* (2nd ed.). Wiley-Blackwell.

8 SLOWING DOWN TO BEGIN WRITING

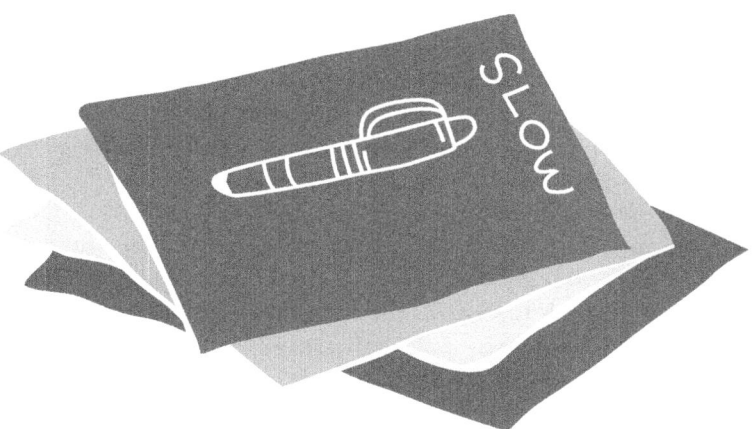

The eighth chapter, Slowing Down to Begin Writing, focuses on distancing ourselves from our busy lives to create space for writing. Just like with data analysis, writing in qualitative research requires thinking time, which means we need to remove physical and mental distractions to create room for creativity. The chapter covers how to begin writing, what challenges the researcher will encounter, and how to address them in the writing process. The "busy mind" is addressed, and suggestions for disengaging and freeing ourselves from the busyness are introduced as opportunities to create space and overcome writing challenges. The steps for the breaking the habit of busyness meditation are included in the chapter. The chapter finishes with the conclusion, key takeaways, and reflection questions. A section to capture indispensable *Mindful Memos* is included with a summary of the practice.

THE BUSY MIND

This chapter focuses on the busy mind and how it can complicate or cloud the creative process required for writing in qualitative research. The busy mind is often referred to as the monkey mind in meditation. It is natural for one's mind to race, especially during the meditation practice. No matter how experienced the meditator, they will experience the monkey mind. Bai (2015) shared that "[w]e are so deeply conditioned, as it were, to run on the monkey mind program, that it is very difficult for us to switch off the program" (p. 144). We cannot force our minds to not have thoughts because it is the nature of the mind to do so. Often, when we sit down and begin our practice, we notice our active monkey mind. Our thoughts move around like a monkey jumping from tree to tree and branch to branch. Fundamentally, the mind has a hard time sitting still. I am sure you have experienced it at several points over your engagement with the practices in this book.

We don't want to avoid the busy mind, but instead find a way to rein it in. The key is being able to tamper down the busyness in a way that leads to focus and creativity. Think about a surgeon. She might be thinking about her partner, what will be for dinner later on, or her weekend plans as she scrubs in for surgery. But as soon as she enters into the operating room, it is vital her mind be in the present moment. If she finds herself still jumping from thought to thought, it will impact her ability to perform her job, which in most cases has someone's life on the line. Therefore, relying on the breathwork skills presented in this chapter, we will be able to tame the monkey mind and prepare for the important task at hand.

The particular kind of breathwork that helps us navigate a busy mind is the box breath or four-square breath. This meditation practice is more intentionally focused on the breath, where you breathe in for a number of counts and out for a number of counts while holding the breath in-between. Athletes, military personnel, nurses, and anyone else who experiences stress in their jobs can benefit from using this approach. We will cover the step-by-step process later in the chapter.

In terms of research, scholars have investigated the ways in which meditation and the box breath can be a useful tool for persons dealing with anxiety and stress that stem from a busy mind. Specifically, Wisner (2013) conducted a study of high school students who participated in an 8-week meditation program. The findings demonstrated the benefits of adopting a meditation practice to navigate anxiety and stress along with the busy mind. Eliuk and Chorney (2017) also explored how students in secondary education can use mindfulness training to combat the monkey mind. Grade competition, perfection desires, and parental pressures cultivate a monkey mind, which leads to added stress and anxiety. Mindfulness training in the classroom was used to work through and overcome the monkey mind.

UNHOOKING FROM BUSYNESS TO BEGIN WRITING

Writing requires focus, yet enough openness to remain creative. If you find yourself sitting down to write with a busy mind, putting thoughts on paper will become difficult. We have to learn to disengage from a busy mind or monkey mind not only to begin the writing process, but also to remain engaged and present for a period of time with writing.

In some ways, the process of writing is the equivalent to Csikszentmihalyi's (1975) concept of flow. According to Csikszentmihalyi (1991), flow is a psychological state, where people are in their groove or in the zone. It is where people perform the task at hand at their peak ability, and because of that, everything seems to fall into place (1991). One must be in an active state to experience flow, so relaxing on a couch is not a time when flow can be experienced. The idea is to be fully committed and involved in an activity that you are passionate about, where you become so immersed that nothing is on your mind other than what you are doing in that space in time. It is an active state of awareness of being in the present moment, similar to what we experience when we are meditating, but different. The mind is focused and aware, but the activity is what got you there, not a guided meditation.

Both meditation and a state of flow can work together and should not be competing with or struggling against one another. Getting into a state of flow is where the magic happens in writing. This state is where you can write easily, where nothing distracts you, and where the words just materialize. To separate from the busy mind to begin writing, we can rely on our breaking the habit of busyness meditation and breathing techniques presented in this chapter.

POTENTIAL WRITING CHALLENGES

Challenges are undeniably inherent in the writing process, but we need to learn to accept and work through them. I had some predicaments while writing this book. Some chapters came so easily I could barely type fast enough to get my thoughts on paper. However, other chapters slogged on, which is when the busyness bug crept in, and I felt like I had to just get through it. This was not effective and ended up stifling my writing process. So, what did I do? I took the exact same advice I am offering in this book to get through the murky sections. In fact, by slowing down, not rushing, and engaging in my personal meditation practice, I was able to rejuvenate enthusiasm and move forward.

The next section will cover some of the challenges you may encounter or questions you should address during the writing process, which include how to get started, what to include, and how to strengthen the theoretical and practical implications.

How to Get Started. Similar to data analysis, just getting started can be a difficult part of the writing process. However, setting up your environment with an adequate block of time is the first step in getting started. Like the environment you created to begin data analysis, you will adopt the same approach here, although the elements you incorporate may be different.

The first step is to decide what time of day you write best. Is it the morning, late at night, or after lunch? This time of day may be the same as when you prefer to analyze data, or it may be different. The second step is to create an inviting environment where creativity is welcomed. Would you prefer to be at a coffee shop, where the ambient noise with others working creates inspiration? Do you want to be on your couch, at home, or in the office? Do you need acoustic or electronic music playing, or is silence best? What about the temperature? Should it be warm or cool? Would you like to sip on a cup of coffee or tea (which might be an ideal fit if you are working at a coffee shop)? Or maybe caffeine makes you too jittery, so you stick with water? How about snacks? Do you prefer to eat a little along the way or stop for a food break?

The key is to create an environment that cultivates creativity and insight, which is a bit different than the type of environment needed for data analysis. Specifically, data analysis required you to set up an environment to access the left, more analytical side of your brain. And here, with writing, you need to access the right, more creative side of your brain. Given the differences, a special environment may be required. For me, I prefer to conduct data analysis at my office, with peace and quiet. However, for writing, I often find a local coffee shop the most inspiring environment for me.

Therefore, before we even begin writing, we need to slow down and ask ourselves: What do I need? Oftentimes, we do not always take the time to focus on our own needs, putting others before ourselves. However, to be able to immerse ourselves in our data and develop the story that best represents the lived experiences of our participants, we need to slow down and check-in. One of the ways we can do that is to tap into our five senses, which we explored in Chapter 5. You will want to pause and take some time to think through the needs of each one of your senses to develop creativity. Below is an exercise for you to review what is needed for the five senses to create the best writing environment to help you get started. The questions included here are simply suggestions for you to craft the optimum writing environment. Use these as a jumping-off point as you dive into what would be needed to get creativity flowing.

USING OUR FIVE SENSES TO DEVELOP CREATIVITY

1. Sight: Should the space you are working in be bright or dark? Do you prefer natural light, bright light, or low light?

2. Smell: Do you like to have a candle burning? Or do you prefer to have no scent, as it might become distracting?
3. Sound: Should your space be quiet or loud? Do you prefer music? If so, what kind?
4. Taste: Do you want to snack along the way? If so, what kind? Do you prefer to stay hydrated or caffeinated, or both?
5. Touch: Do you want to be warm or cold? What kind of chair do you want to be in? Do you prefer to stand? Do you want to be alone or surrounded by strangers?

One last note about getting started is related to knowing when to step away. You might sit down to write and have a great session, where you knock out whole sections of a manuscript. However, there might be times when you position yourself to write, and nothing comes out. It is in these moments that we must be willing to step away. Trying to struggle through writer's block will not work. Instead, engage in meditation or find another way to relinquish it, so ultimately you are able to create space in your mind that will help you get refreshed for the next writing session.

Slowing down and creating space is how we generate creativity, which almost seems counterintuitive. Most would think that speedily jumping from one task to the next is how we tackle writing, but that is not true. When we take time to slow down, we are able to think deeper and harvest our creativity. For example, the idea for this book was envisioned while I was on a beach vacation reading a nonacademic, fiction book. Somehow, as I was sitting there, relaxing, and reading, the idea of using mindfulness as a qualitative research tool popped into my mind. I have had an active meditation practice for over a decade, so I had ample experience with the practices in this book, in addition to years of qualitative research experience. However, blending the two never occurred to me until that moment. Therefore, if you are at a standstill in your writing process, give yourself permission to step away and take a break.

What Data to Include. The second challenge that a qualitative researcher may face is what data to include. I will be the first to admit that cutting or not including all the incredible data that emerge from a qualitative research project can be an arduous task. Inevitably, because of page number limitations, qualitative researchers will be faced with having to decide what data to include, which is easier said than done. However, I offer a practical recommendation, as well as share how slowing down can aid with figuring out what data to include.

In terms of the practical suggestion, I keep track of who is included and how many times they have been quoted in my findings section. I have a list of my participants off to the side while I am writing findings. As soon as I quote a person, I make a hashmark near their name. I continue with this until the findings section is complete. This process ensures every participant is included in the findings. It also assists in confirming that one or two participants were not overused. Unsurprisingly, certain participants will be more loquacious than others or more succinct with what they share. I find it hard not to use these participants' quotes several times over the course of the findings. However, it is imperative that findings represent everyone's experience and not just the few who were the most verbose. Therefore, keeping track can be extremely beneficial.

Relying on the meditation presented in this chapter can also be advantageous when trying to decide what and how much data to include. There is a certain level of contentment experienced when you spend time concentrating on the breath. Even more so, when you calm the mind, and not jump from one thought to the next, your thoughts become more focused. When we have a corpus of data in front of us, our minds become cluttered, which feels stifling. However, if we stop, slow down, and focus on the breath using the exercises in this chapter, we are able to gain clarity in our data. In doing so, we can identify the data that ought to be included in the findings.

How to Strengthen Implications.   The third challenge addressed in this chapter deals with the implications of the research project. This can oftentimes be one of the hardest tasks that any qualitative researcher encounters. Ultimately, this is the challenge to answer the question of "So what?" The hurdle is finding both theoretical and, in most cases, practical implications for the study. Not all fields require the practical aspect, but our field does. The majority of public relations and strategic communication journals encourage authors to include implications that can be used in practice based on the insights from the study. Sometimes implications are easy to find, but other times we must be willing to explore, which makes this a challenge in the writing process.

From my experience, many graduate students struggle with the "so what" question. I teach a qualitative research methods course at the doctoral level in my college, and the class attracts students across campus. I often find that almost all students grapple with the broader impact of their research. They might collect rich data and perform rigorous analysis, but when it comes to writing the discussion, more could be done to strengthen the theoretical (and practical) implications. In other words, the writing becomes a written report versus an opportunity for discovery (Charmaz, 2007).

To enhance the implications using practical tools, we have a couple of different options. First, we can revisit the data and conduct further analysis. Second, participating in a few peer debriefing sessions might be helpful. I personally have found great success in talking through findings with someone else, especially if they are a subject matter expert. For example, a colleague and I worked on a case study to investigate a crisis within an organization. I provided a coding tree of the insights to her ahead of our meeting. When we met, we discussed each of the emergent themes, and she was able to strengthen some and collapse others, which enhanced the implications of our study. Third, revisiting the literature to see what potential gaps the study is fulfilling might also be a beneficial approach. Fourth, I suggest having a document open or a spiral notebook on hand while writing the findings to capture discussion implications in real time. Inevitably, insights will come to mind while immersed in the writing process, and you don't want to forget these. Fifth, ambiguity and uncertainty need to be embraced as a means to cultivate creativity (Charmaz, 2007). Ultimately, we must learn to trust the writing process (Charmaz, 2007).

Nevertheless, beyond the aforementioned suggestions, relying on the breathwork to calm and quiet the mind is a great way to see things more clearly. When taking a moment to pause and participate in a meditation, we can slow down. In slowing down, we are able to see things a bit more clearly. Even if you simply participate in a round of box breathing, this can often be enough to silence the mind so that the implications of your research become clearer. If we find ourselves on a busy path while writing, we may miss some of the great insights garnered from the study. Slowing down helps us see small details that eventually end up being something big in the end.

THE PRACTICE: BREAKING THE HABIT OF BUSYNESS MEDITATION

The practice we are about to embark on features a meditation that includes two breathing techniques. This two-part meditation is useful in calming the busy mind and helping us to tune into our present experiences. When we quiet the mind, we are able to cultivate space that can enhance our creative abilities, which is needed when we write.

In many cases, it takes 20 or 25 minutes for the mind to settle, which is the time frame for this chapter's meditation. We have worked to develop our skills so that we are able to sit for longer periods of time. But you shouldn't be concerned about or focused on time. Our goal is simply to accept what is going on and not judge it. If you often experience a monkey mind while meditating, just notice the busyness. When you are swept away by thoughts, pull yourself back using the following breathing practices that we are going to explore in our meditation.

When you experience thoughts, know that you are not doing anything wrong; it just means you are experiencing a normal, human reaction. Come back to the breath with patience and understanding when you notice yourself being wrapped up in thought. Recognize that thoughts, mental activity—possibly even discomfort—are all part of the meditation experience. Let there be sound, let there be emotion, let everything you are experiencing in that moment simply be. When we learn to observe our experience without exercising a judgment about whether it is right or wrong, this is when we are mastering our practice, moving into becoming a more advanced practitioner.

Start by finding a quiet place to sit and then setting your alarm for 20 to 25 minutes. Be sure you are in a comfortable, seated position where you can remain focused but relaxed. Check-in with your posture to ensure you are sitting up straight but not too rigid. Find a comfortable, balanced position that is easy to sustain. Let your neck, shoulders, and forehead feel soft. Allow your hands to feel heavy, and let your attention rest on your breath.

We are going to begin by focusing on a practice called the box breath. You will begin by breathing in for four counts, holding the breath for four counts, exhaling for four counts, and then holding the exhale for four counts. Again, breath in for one, two, three, four. Hold for one, two, three, four. Exhale for one, two, three, four. Hold for one, two, three, four. Repeat the full cycle of box breathing four times. Then pause, and resume a slow, natural breath.

The breath flows in, and the breath flows out. One breath at time, not trying to jump ahead to the next one, but sitting and relaxing in each breath. You can now transition to counting the breaths to quiet the busy mind. Breathe all the way in and then breathe all the way out and count one. Breathe all the way in and all the way out and count two. Once you have been able to focus on three to four full cycles of breath, concentration continues to deepen. Count all the way up to 10 if needed. Then you will begin again, counting each breath as it comes and goes.

Whenever you notice that your attention has shifted, bring your attention back to the breath. Part of this practice is to learn noticing when we have become distracted, and then coming back. Having a busy mind is a natural part of sitting, so there is no need to get frustrated with ourselves for being unfocused. What is most important is the attitude you develop toward the busy mind. Each time you find yourself distracted by a feeling, thought, or sensation, see it as an offering to return to awareness with patience and acceptance. Always come back with a level of friendliness toward the self. Simply notice where the mind is and return to the breath by counting each one. Again, breathe all the way in and all the way out and count one. Breathe all the way in and all the way out and count two. Continue to move between both breathing practices for the remainder of the session.

Now, slowly feel into the sensations of your body. Move your hands and fingers. Come back to the sounds in the room. Take one last deep breath, and when you are ready, open your eyes.

The breaking the habit of busyness meditation that incorporates the two breathing techniques will be your practice for the next 2 weeks. I realize our meditations have gotten longer and longer, but I encourage you to commit time each day to the full 20 to 25 minutes. At the end of each practice, spend time capturing your *Mindful Memos*. You will want to write down your thoughts and feelings about the practice as well as your observations about the busy mind and how it may (or may not) be shifting over the course of the 2 weeks. The *Mindful Memos* is how we can see ourselves change in addition to experiencing our change.

This meditation can be used before every writing session. It can also be intertwined into the moments in your life when you are feeling overwhelmed or find life hectic. Using the breath to create a pause is a wonderful way to create space. In addition, the breathing techniques introduced in the meditation can be great tools to rely on at any moment in time, not necessarily while sitting in a meditation. For example, you might use the box breath the next time you are stuck in traffic or receive a call with bad news. Or you might count to 10 using the breath before your next big presentation. With either approach, you will be able to relax the mind and minimize restless thoughts.

CONCLUSION

This chapter focused on learning how to slow down to begin writing. To write, we need mental space and to find a way to calm our monkey minds. You might need other elements to cultivate a creative writing space—suggestions were made in the chapter. Also discussed were the ways to get started writing, how to decide what to include, and the ways in which the theoretical and practical implications can be strengthened. Two breathing techniques were introduced and explained: the box breath and counting. In learning to slow down, we are able to enhance our creativity and prepare for the writing process.

KEY TAKEAWAYS

- This chapter focused on your busy mind and how it can complicate or cloud the creative process required for writing in qualitative research. In meditation, the busy mind is often referred to as the monkey mind.

- Despite the times in which you have experienced a busy mind, know that it is a natural occurrence.

- The particular kind of breathwork that helps us navigate a busy mind is the box breath or four-square breath.

- Challenges are inherent in the writing process, but slowing down can help us overcome those challenges.

- The breathing techniques introduced in the meditation can be great tools to rely on at any moment in time, not necessarily while sitting in a meditation.

REFLECTION QUESTIONS

- How often do you feel the monkey mind creeping into your everyday activities? When do you experience it during meditation?

- Have you considered what your environment needs to look like to begin writing? Share your ideal writing environment.

- What excites you about the writing process?

- Have you ever experienced writer's block? What was that experience like, and how did you get through it?

THE 2-WEEK PRACTICE: BREAKING THE BUSYNESS HABIT MEDITATION

Your practice for the next 2 weeks focuses on two different breathwork practices to break out of the habit of being busy experiencing the monkey mind. The first practice is the box breath, which focuses on breathing in, pausing, breathing out, and pausing all to a count of four. The second practice is counting breaths up to 10 and then repeating. Both practices are useful in calming the busy mind, which is a reflection of our current culture that tends to champion and award those who are the busiest. But constantly being busy results in having a monkey mind that jumps from one thought to the next with no space for rest. To write, we need to cultivate quiet, and this meditation will help us get there. Dedicate time each day to the breaking the busyness habit meditation. Be sure to record your *Mindful Memos* following each meditation so you can witness what happens when you work on taming the monkey mind.

Mindful Memos

_____

_____

_____

_____

_____

_____

_____

_____

_____

_____

_____

_____

_____

_____

_____

_____

_____

_____

_____

_____

_____

_____

_____

_____

_____

_____

_____

_____

REFERENCES

Bai, H. (2015). Peace with the earth: Animism and contemplative ways. *Cultural Studies of Science Education*, *10*(1), 135–147. https://doi.org/10.1007/s11422-01 3-9501

Charmaz, K. (2007). Tensions in qualitative research. *Sociologisk Forskning*, *44*(3), 76–85.

Csikszentmihalyi, M. (1975). Play and intrinsic rewards. *Journal of Humanistic Psychology*, *15*(3), 41–63. https://doi.org/10.1177/002216787501500306

Csikszentmihalyi, M. (1990). *Flow: The psychology of optimal experience*. Harper & Row.

Eliuk, K., & Chorney, D. (2017). Calming the monkey mind. *International Journal of Higher Education*, *6*(2). 1–7. https://doi.org/10.5430/ijhe.v6n2p1

Wisner, B. L. (2013). Less stress, less drama, and experiencing monkey mind: Benefits and challenges of a school-based meditation program for adolescents. *School Social Work Journal*, *38*(1), 49–63.

9 CONCLUSION

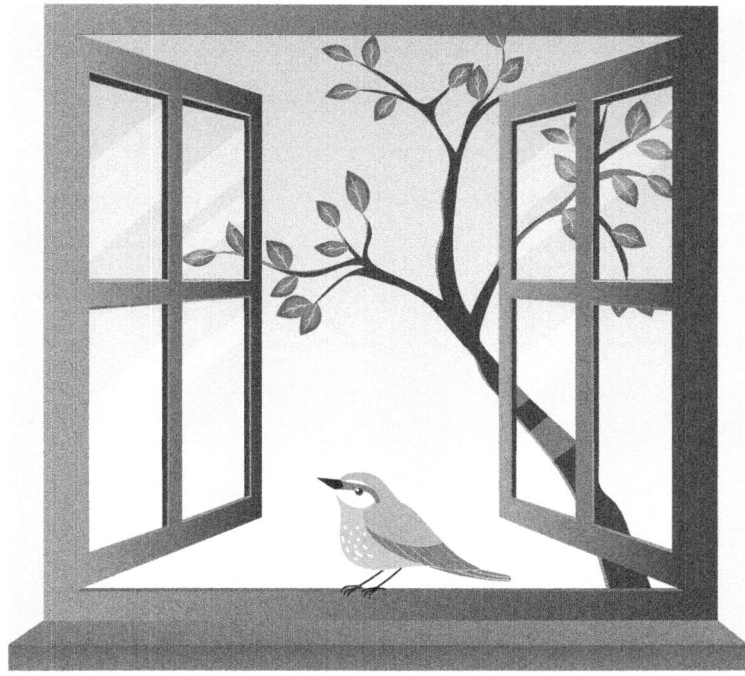

As we wrap up our time together, I want you to reflect on what you have learned over each of the preceding chapters. Take some time to revisit your *Mindful Memos* from each chapter, working chronologically across the entries. What did you learn about yourself? How have you changed? How has your view of the qualitative research process shifted? Capture these observations and others in the following *Mindful Memos* section.

Mindful Memos

THE MINDFUL QUALITATIVE RESEARCHER

Being a mindful qualitative researcher (MQR) encompasses various skills and characteristics that were covered in this book. The MQR engages in purposeful self-reflexivity and explores the researcher self at various points in a study. Labeling and walking into a research study with a strong set of beliefs is at a minimum limited, and if possible, avoided, because the MQR knows how this will detract from the current study. The MQR always approaches each new study with a beginner's mind, seeing each new project with fresh eyes. Perfectionism is replaced with relaxation and play for the MQR—the goal is to encourage playfulness and foster creativity. The MQR exerts empathy, compassion, and understanding for the self and participants. For the MQR, curiosity underpins every phase of the research process, and there is a willingness to take risks when necessary, even if the risks are outside of one's comfort zone. MQRs have an intentionality around the research processes, balancing organizational procedures with being open to the emergent design. The MQR knows the ideal environment for data analysis and writing, which is discovered through personal exploration and awareness. Most importantly, the MQR is willing to retreat and rejuvenate to create space in the mind. The intentional space generates an acute attention for the research process that could have been overlooked when the mind was filled with commotion.

Over the course of this book, I hope you witnessed how your mind expanded with the newly found space. In creating space, we are able to prepare ourselves for whatever might occur during any phase of a qualitative study, which strengthens our research abilities.

THE PRACTICES

Each one of the chapters in this book introduced a specific practice that could be used to navigate an aspect of qualitative research. In addition, the length in which we sat in meditation increased as the book progressed, since you were strengthening your capacity for engagement in the present moment. The following paragraphs summarize the practices that were introduced and explored in each chapter.

In **Chapter 2**, we discussed the listening meditation as a means to explore the researcher self. The listening to sounds meditation was a 10-minute meditation that focused on hearing all of the sounds around us, teaching us to pay close attention to sounds in our space that we might have missed.

This meditation also helped us get out of our own heads and into the present moment, so we don't get wrapped up in old narratives and stories about ourselves.

In **Chapter 3**, the body scan was introduced. The body scan meditation was a 10 to 15 minute meditation that allowed us to explore feelings and sensations in the body, moving part by part from the head to the toes. This meditation is helpful in developing the beginner's mind as a way to prepare for interviews and navigate issues that may arise while interviewing.

Chapter 4 covered the loving-kindness meditation, which was a 10 to 15 minute meditation to practice prior to conducting focus groups. This practice prepared us to work with others in a group setting by developing loving-kindness first toward ourselves, and second to those around us. The meditation focused on repeating specific phrases that demonstrate care and kindness.

In **Chapter 5**, we took our practice to the streets, per se, and explored the walking meditation to observe our five senses. This 15 to 20 minute meditation was about awakening all of the senses to prepare for the research setting, specifically for when we immerse ourselves into a context via participant observation or ethnographic research. This meditation is one of the most active ones we explored since we were literally walking and observing our entire environment using the five senses.

For **Chapter 6**, we covered the noting meditation to help with data management and participated in the practice for 15 to 20 minutes for each sit. The noting meditation focused on riding through and simply noting thoughts and emotions arising during the practice. Although this practice was presented as a tool for dealing with data management, it can be incredibly helpful at many points in the research process.

In **Chapter 7**, the open awareness meditation was covered as a tool to navigate data analysis. The open awareness meditation was practiced for 20 to 25 minutes, and its purpose was to expand the mind by building on and combining many of the practices in the earlier chapters. Specifically, the practice allowed the meditator to move from the breath to sounds to the body to thoughts and feelings and finally to whatever might present itself in the present moment.

Chapter 8 was focused on slowing down to begin writing and discussed suggestions for unhooking from busyness as an opportunity to create space and overcome writing challenges. The steps for the breaking the habit of busyness meditation were included in the chapter. The 20 to 25 minute practice focused on two breathing techniques. Specifically, the chapter covered the box breath and the counting of breaths to slow down and create space.

COMMITTING TO THE PRACTICES

Continue to revisit these practices throughout your qualitative research projects. You may find that you prefer certain practices over others or that all are necessary for each phase of a study. I encourage you to make these practices your own and to be creative with how you integrate them into your research process and life in general.

Remember that we have to be continually engaged with a meditation practice to make it useful in research. For example, you cannot pick up a 50-pound dumbbell and attempt to do 10 curls if you have never lifted weights in your life. Same goes for meditation—if you haven't been prioritizing a daily practice, sitting and focusing for 20 minutes or even 10 minutes will be incredibly difficult. By this point, you have worked hard to strengthen your mind in ways that you might not have done before. Therefore, consider keeping the meditation practices active over the coming days and years, so that they become part of your daily routine and part of the fabric of who you are. In doing so, you may find yourself more peaceful, curious, nonreactant, and open to all of life's many experiences.

A CLOSING WITH GRATITUDE

I hope you have noticed by this point that the practices introduced in the book are incredibly helpful in the research process, but they are also tools to navigate and engage with throughout our everyday lives. You should congratulate yourself for what you have accomplished and gained over the course of the weeks associated with reading this book. This is the beginning of a wonderful journey into personal awareness and a deeper connection to the self. Thank you for joining me, and I wish you the best in your future endeavors. Be well.

INDEX